First Episode Psychosis

T0286578

Kathy J Aitchison, BM, BCh, MA, MRCPsych
Institute of Psychiatry,
Department of Psychological Medicine,
London, UK

Karena Meehan, MB, BCh, BAO, MRCP, MRCPsych
Institute of Psychiatry,
Department of Psychological Medicine,
London, UK

Robin M Murray, MD, DSc, FRCP, FRCPsych
Institute of Psychiatry,
Department of Psychological Medicine,
London, UK

MARTIN DUNITZ

© Martin Dunitz 1999

First published in the United Kingdom in 1999 by

Martin Dunitz Ltd
The Livery House
7-9 Pratt Street
London NW1 0AE

A CIP record for this book is available from the British Library.

ISBN 1-85317-435-1

Distributed in the United States by:
Blackwell Science Inc.
Commerce Place, 350 Main Street
Malden, MA 02148, USA
Tel: 1-800-215-1000

Distributed in Canada by:
Login Brothers Book Company
324 Salteaux Crescent
Winnipeg, Manitoba, R3J 3T2
Canada
Tel: 204-224-4068

Distributed in Brazil by:
Ernesto Reichmann Distribuidora de Livros, Ltda
Rua Coronel Marques 335, Tatuape 03440-000
Sao Paulo,
Brazil

Composition by Scribe Design, Gillingham, Kent, UK
Printed and bound in Italy.
Cover illustration by Janet Powick, a professional artist who has experienced schizophrenia.

Contents

Kathy J Aitchison is currently a Research Fellow in the Section of Clinical Neuropharmacology, Department of Psychological Medicine, at the Institute of Psychiatry, London. She graduated in Physiological Sciences from Oxford University and trained in medicine at Oxford University Clinical Medical School, and in psychiatry at The Bethlem Royal and Maudsley Hospitals, London.

Karena Meehan attended University College Galway in Ireland, where she obtained her medical degree before training in internal medicine in Dublin and becoming a Member of the Royal College of Physicians. Completing her psychiatry training at the Maudsley Hospital, London, she subsequently held a research appointment at the associated Institute of Psychiatry, where the focus area of her research was on the epidemiology, course and treatment of first episode psychosis. She continues to practice as an Honorary Clinical Research Psychiatrist at the Maudsley Hospital and the Department of Psychological Medicine at the Institute of Psychiatry, in London.

Robin M Murray has been Professor of the Joint Department of Psychological Medicine of King's College School of Medicine and Dentistry and the Institute of Psychiatry since 1989. Prior to that, he was Dean of the Institute of Psychiatry. Between 1994–1996 he was President of the Association of European Psychiatrists. He was one of the first to propose that schizophrenia was a neurodevelopmental disorder and has carried out extensive neuroimaging studies of schiz- ophrenia as well as epidemiological studies into the role of early cerebral insults as risk factors for the disorder. Professor Murray also runs two clinical teams; a District Unit which provides psychiatric services and the National Psychoses Unit, which is based at the Bethlem Royal Hospital. Those with psychotic illnesses who have not responded to conventional treatment are referred here from all over England.

Acknowledgements

The following have made valuable contributions to this book in various ways: Miss B Greenall, Mr P Goldacre, Drs D and N Beer, Dr and Mrs A Kinnear, Mr D Taylor, Dr P Hayward, Dr R Kemp, Dr G Kuperberg, Prof SA Checkley, Prof C Kumar, Prof M Birchwood, Prof PD McGorry, and Dr W Sellwood. We would like to thank any others who have offered us support in this work. We would also like to thank our publishers, particularly our editor Yasmin Khan-Chowdhury.

Dedication

To all who have experienced a first psychotic episode.

Why focus on the first episode?

1

In recent years, increased attention has focused on the first presentation and early course of psychosis. The main reason for this is the realization that treatment is least effective in those patients who have been psychotic for many years. The obvious implication is that closer attention should be paid to patients during the period when the vulnerability to psychosis is first expressed, in the hope that intervention at this point may prevent irreversible neurobiological and social changes.

As early as 1927 Harry Stack Sullivan said of schizophrenia, 'I feel certain that any incipient cases might be arrested before the efficient contact with reality is completely suspended, and a long stay in institutions made necessary'.[1] Subsequently, Cameron wrote of the value of a preventive approach to schizophrenia, describing the importance of 'the detection of very early disorder to prevent later serious ill health'.[2] Such views have been echoed by many recent authorities who believe that early diagnosis and treatment may minimize or even prevent the

Table 1
Treatment lag in studies of first-episode schizophrenia.

Study	Setting	n	Definition	Treatment lag
Beiser et al[7]	Vancouver	72	DSM-III	56 weeks
Birchwood et al[10]	Birmingham	128	ICD-9	30 weeks
Johnstone et al[6]	London	253	ICD-9	28% < 8 weeks
				26% > 52 weeks
Loebel et al[5]	New York	70	RDC	52 weeks
McGorry & Singh[11]	Melbourne	60	DSM-III-R	74 weeks

From Birchwood et al.[10]

devastating psychological and social disturbances that result from continued florid psychosis.[3,4]

The importance of early treatment

Much evidence suggests that most patients who present to psychiatrists with their first episode of psychosis have, in fact, been ill for a considerable period (Table 1). For instance, one group in New York found that their patients had suffered psychotic symptoms for an average of 1 year before treatment started.[5] Other research groups in the UK,[6] Canada,[7] Australia[8] and Germany[9] have reported a similarly long interval between the onset of psychotic symptoms and the initiation of appropriate treatment. In the Northwick Park study,[6] the delay before treatment started was longer than 1 year in about a quarter of patients with their first episode of schizophrenia. Furthermore, delay was associated with increasing complications such as severe behavioural disturbance, family difficulties and life-threatening behaviour. The New York group also described an increased risk of life-threatening crises, due either to aggression or suicidal behaviour;[5] substance abuse, either as a cause or an attempt to self medicate, may further complicate the picture. The delay for affective psychosis may be shorter than for schizophrenia,[7] though the evidence is conflicting.

Such delays bring obvious distress to patients and their relatives. The patient is usually frightened and may feel extremely isolated from family and friends. When, as is commonly the case, the first episode occurs in adolescence or early adulthood the result can be particularly disruptive. Potentially even more important, however, is the question of whether delay before treatment with antipsychotics actually worsens the long-term outcome. Many psychiatrists believe that the severity of psychotic illness has attenuated over the twentieth century, and that fewer patients have deteriorated to a chronic incapacitated state since the introduction of antipsychotics.[12] Although it is impossible to single out antipsychotics as the sole cause of this change, the temporal relationship is suggestive.

The Northwick Park study reported that those patients taking longer than 1 year to access services (a quarter of their sample) showed a three-fold increase in relapse rate over the following 2 years, compared with those with a briefer duration of untreated psychosis.[6]

Untreated illness emerged as the strongest predictor of relapse irrespective of the use of maintenance medication. The New York group also noted that those patients who had had positive psychotic symptoms for long periods without antipsychotic medication had a slower and less complete recovery, and increased subsequent risk of relapse, than those who received prompt treatment.[5] It is difficult to exclude the possibility that the former group had a more insidious onset than the latter and, of course, it is well known that patients with an insidious onset fare worse.

Nevertheless Wyatt, who reviewed the literature,[13] concluded that delay in treating psychosis might indeed worsen the long-term outcome; he went on to suggest that untreated psychosis is biologically toxic and contributes to long-term morbidity.[14] Thus, while the evidence to date does not conclusively demonstrate that early intervention with antipsychotics can alter the natural history of psychosis, many clinicians believe that it is only fair to give patients the benefit of the doubt.

Early detection and referral

One of the barriers to early treatment is that relatives often fail to realize that the sufferer is ill, attributing the changed behaviour to, for example, adolescent problems or to the stress of college or work. Unusual or even bizarre behaviour in adolescents is less likely to attract attention or cause comment than in other age groups, and this may further exacerbate treatment delay. Relatives may also deny the seriousness of the behaviour through fear of mental illness and its stigma. Even when families recognize the illness, their difficulties may be only just beginning; the Northwick Park group reported that patients and their relatives often had made many contacts with services before receiving appropriate help![6]

Since general practitioners are most frequently the first point of contact for patients and their families[15] it is vital that those in primary care can recognize the early symptoms of psychosis. Social services and, perhaps surprisingly, the police may also be very helpful to families in getting treatment,[16] and deserve to be included in any educational campaign about psychosis.

Thus, factors that can lead to treatment delays include:

- fears about the consequences of having a mental disorder
- difficulties in gaining access to mental health services
- poor screening by primary care health professionals
- inexact diagnosis by mental health professionals

General practitioners, or others who make first contact, need to have access to a psychiatric service to which they can confidently refer those they suspect of having a first episode of psychosis, in the knowledge that they will receive prompt assessment and appropriate care. While this may seem obvious, many standard psychiatric services are more geared to the ongoing care of chronic relapsing patients than the treatment of the newly ill; indeed, the facilities such services provide may be inappropriate, and the other users frightening, for the young, first-onset patient. It is therefore vital that the initial assessment of a first episode of psychosis should (a) be prompt, (b) be comprehensive and (c) occur in a user-friendly environment.

Various strategies have been proposed to minimize treatment delay:

- education focusing on community and voluntary agencies likely to encounter psychosis (college counsellors, homeless agencies, etc)
- intensive training of primary care professionals in the recognition of early psychosis

- rapid access to specialist opinion
- early assignment of a key-worker to facilitate engagement with mental health services
- early treatment in a low-stigma setting—for example through a home-treatment team

Treatment

The treatment itself should maximize therapeutic benefit and minimize side-effects since this initial period is likely to set the tone of the subsequent relationship between patient and the services. For example, immediate prescription of a high dose of a 'typical' antipsychotic (for example 20 mg of haloperidol within 24 hours) may induce a severe dystonic reaction with subsequent (justified) distrust of the clinician. Instead, there has been much interest in the work of those such as McEvoy *et al*,[17] who found that low 'neuroleptic threshold' doses (an average of 3.4 mg haloperidol) led to symptomatic recovery in acutely ill, recent-onset patients; higher doses did not quicken treatment response.

Psychological treatment should be part of both initial and continuing care[18] (see Chapters 7 and 8).

The focus of care should be not only on inducing a rapid remission but also on the re-integration of the patient back into his/her community, with continued monitoring to maximize recovery and prevent relapse. Indeed, a first-onset service should have a *psychosis register* of all referrals of psychotic patients to ensure that those who have made contact do not drop out of care.

Possible long-term benefits of early treatment

Birchwood and McMillan[4] point out that the majority of the social, psychological and biological deterioration shown by psychotic patients occurs in the first 5 years—the *critical period.* Indeed, Birchwood *et al* suggest that the early phase of psychosis is both formative and predictive of long-term outcome.[19] Perhaps, therefore, it would be wiser to try to prevent early deterioration rather than continue to spend the vast bulk of healthcare resources on the care of patients with established psychosis who may be relatively treatment resistant. Indeed, some preliminary evidence does suggest that putting more resources into the intensive treatment of early psychosis may lead not only to more rapid remission of psychosis, but also to better long-term outcome and thus lower long-term costs.[10,20] The possible benefits of such early treatment include:

- earlier recovery
- less disruption to social and occupational life
- better long-term outcome
- decreased hospitalization
- lower long-term costs of care

Relapse can be expected in 40–60% of patients within 2 years of first treatment.[21,22] Each relapse results in an increased chance of treatment resistance and deterioration in social functioning. Maintenance medication is thought to offer some protection but the doses used should avoid impairment of social function (see Chapter 5).

There has been little research on the early psychosocial adjustment to psychosis, but it is an issue of major importance. This is a period carrying a high risk for suicide—hardly surprising in view of the enormous change in attitudes and expectations engendered by both the experience of psychotic symptoms and by a diagnosis of major mental illness. Problems of low self-regard and hopelessness,[23] together with social stigma and loss of status, make

this a high-risk period for self-injurious behaviour.

Long-term prospective studies of cohorts of first-onset psychosis patients are extremely rare; an important study from Madras reviewed 90 such patients monthly for 10 years,[24] with few lost to follow up, and found positive and negative symptoms stabilized by the second year, affecting 25% of the sample, with no significant further deterioration or evidence of substitution of positive for negative symptoms. The lack of further decline after 3–5 years has also been shown by other studies.[25,26]

Summary

The last decade has seen a rapid development in our understanding of psychosis. We believe that this knowledge is now feeding into the clinical arena, bringing new hope to our patients and their families. Maximization of the benefits of the new pharmacological and psychosocial treatments requires a focus on the patient from their first contact with the services.

In particular, an approach designed to detect and treat this patient group at the earliest possible stage may offer the possibility of preventing the development of some of the secondary disability and handicap. Patients suffering their first psychotic episode have particular needs. This pocketbook sets out to demonstrate how targeting this group may allow better understanding of their requirements, the development of specialized therapeutic interventions and the prevention or amelioration of subsequent decline in function.

The presentation and assessment of the first psychotic episode

2

The first clinical presentation of psychosis varies greatly from one patient to the next, depending on many factors including age and sex, setting and whether the picture reflects an underlying schizophrenic or affective illness. However, it is often not possible to make the latter distinction immediately. Hence, it is more useful to consider the symptomatology in terms of the main abnormal phenomena seen; this is often a good pointer towards the appropriate therapy, for example the presence of psychotic symptoms suggests the need for an antipsychotic whether or not the eventual diagnosis is likely to be schizophrenia or not.[6] It is important to remember that even symptoms such as hallucinations, which are generally regarded as hallmarks of psychosis, are sometimes experienced by healthy people, for example, when falling asleep or after a bereavement. It is the intensity and persistence of the symptoms as well as their effect on social functioning which suggest that this is the first manifestation of psychosis.

Table 2
Clinical symptoms of psychosis.

Disorders of perception	
hallucinations:	auditory (most common)
	visual
	olfactory
	tactile
	visceral
delusions:	abnormal beliefs; eg nihilistic, grandiose
disorders of the stream of thought:	abnormalities of the amount and speed of thought
disorders of the form of thought:	abnormalities of the way thoughts are linked together
disorders of the possession of thought:	disturbance of the usual awareness that one's thoughts are one's own
Disorders of emotion	
alterations in nature	high or low
alterations in reactivity	labile or blunted
inappropriate	eg inappropriate laughter
Disorders of cognition	
Disorders of insight	
Motor abnormalities	

Similarly, the presentation may vary from insidious to the most acute. Some cases of schizophrenia develop insidiously and on the background of childhood impairments of personality and cognition, so that it is difficult to know when the prodrome of the psychosis, and indeed the psychosis itself, began. Hafner and colleagues have studied the development of psychotic symptoms in great detail and maintain that in such cases, negative symptoms often antedate the positive by several years.[27] Such insidious onsets are particularly ominous and herald a poor prognosis. On the other hand, the more acute onsets tend to herald schizoaffective, manic or drug-induced illnesses with a better outcome.

Paradoxically, the more florid the disturbance and the more obvious the social precipitant, the better is the outcome. The signs and symptoms of psychosis are well described in standard texts,[28,29] but are briefly outlined in Table 2.

Formulation

In first-episode psychosis, as in most psychiatric illness, coming to an appropriate diagnosis is dependent on obtaining a clear history and performing a thorough mental state and physical examination. The details of such an assessment are beyond the scope of this chapter but are given in standard texts.[30] There are no diagnostic blood tests or radiographs, so the clinician's skill in eliciting information is paramount. The first diagnostic task facing the clinician is to distinguish an episode of psychosis from a dauntingly wide range of psychiatric and medical conditions.

Conditions to be excluded

Medical

Physical illnesses which produce psychotic symptoms are relatively unusual, but because of their seriousness, and the potential benefits of appropriate treatment, it is important to identify or exclude them:

- epilepsy (especially temporal lobe epilepsy)
- central nervous system trauma or neoplasm
- HIV infection +/− intracerebral lesion
- encephalitis
- Huntington's disease
- systemic lupus erythematosus
- neurosyphilis
- endocrine disorders such as thyroid or parathyroid disorder, or Cushings disease, Addison's disease or phaeochromocytoma
- metabolic disorders such as B_{12} or folate deficiency, porphyria, chronic hypoglycemia, Wilson's disease

Investigations

In all patients, regular full blood count, electrolyte and urine tests should be carried out. Chest radiographs, liver and thyroid function tests and B_{12} and folate levels may also be appropriate. When the patient is sufficiently calm, magnetic resonance imaging (MRI) of the brain should be carried out (or a computed tomography (CT) scan if MRI is not available), as well as electroencephalography (EEG). Very occasionally, lumbar puncture may be necessary. An electrocardiogram (ECG) should be carried out on anyone in whom cardiac disease is suspected, or if a drug which prolongs the QTc interval is to be used.

Nonmedical

In general, these pose more of a diagnostic problem, in part because psychotic symptoms are often superimposed upon a previous unusual personality, but also because there is no sharp dividing line between psychotic illness and certain personality disorders. Indeed, occasionally it is only after a patient responds well to an antipsychotic that one realizes that behaviour which was initially labelled as secondary to personality disorder was in fact a manifestation of psychosis:

- adolescence turmoil
- schizotypal personality disorder
- borderline personality disorder
- cultural syndromes
- factitious psychosis (rare)

Investigations

Such conditions can only be excluded after a thorough psychiatric and social assessment. This can of course be carried out as part of the general psychosocial assessment which will be required before any of the psychosocial treatments outlined in Chapters 7 and 8 are initiated. It is important to ensure that such assessment includes tests of neuropsychological functioning, although it is probably better to leave this until the patient is able to concentrate, perhaps a few weeks after the initiation of treatment.

The nature of the psychosis

Once it has been ascertained that this is indeed the first presentation of a functional psychosis, the next question is to determine, if possible, which type this illness represents. This will be possible in those cases which present a clear-cut and distinctive picture, but not in others. Therefore, it is often more appropriate to retain the more general term rather than to try and fit a patient inappropriately into a specific category. Indeed, much recent evidence suggests that psychosis is better seen as a continuum of psychopathology.[31]

Those fortunate patients who only have one short episode of psychosis may therefore never progress further than a diagnosis of acute psychosis. In others, the picture will become clearer with time, either later in the first episode or subsequently. The main conditions included under the general term 'functional psychosis' are:

- schizophrenia
- schizoaffective disorder
- affective psychosis: mania, psychotic depression and mixed affective psychosis
- drug-induced psychosis

Some first-episode patients will show symptoms and signs suggestive of schizophrenia but will never quite fit ICD-10 or DSM-IV criteria and therefore will be termed 'schizophreniform', while others will continue to be regarded as having an 'atypical psychosis'; occasional patients will receive a diagnosis of persistent delusional disorder.

It is of particular importance to determine whether the psychotic symptoms are being driven by mood disturbance or by drug abuse.

Mood disorder

The main importance of distinguishing between schizophrenia and affective psychosis lies in whether the patient should receive a mood stabilizer as well as an antipsychotic. Apart from the classic symptoms of mania, symptoms such as irritability, anger and paranoia may be indications for a mood stabilizer. Bizarre mood-congruent delusions or hallucinations are perfectly consistent with a diagnosis of mania, as long as the affective symptoms are present most of the time.

Drug abuse

Both prescribed drugs and drugs of abuse can precipitate the onset of a psychotic episode. Steroids can cause a manic illness in some predisposed individuals. The positive symptoms of schizophrenia can be reproduced by LSD, ecstasy ('E') and amphetamine. Phenylcyclidine (PCP) can cause these as well as apathy, emotional withdrawal and loss of motivation, while many clinicians believe that prolonged heavy abuse of cannabis can induce psychosis. Urine screening should be carried out in all cases of first-episode psychosis. There is some recent evidence that hair analysis, where available, is more accurate and often shows evidence of drug abuse even when this is strenuously denied at first.[32]

Assessment of risk

It is vital to assess the risk of other untoward behaviours, in particular suicide and violence.

Suicide

Some 10–15% of psychotic patients will eventually kill themselves.[33] The risk is greater in the first few years. For example, Van Os *et al*[34] found that 4% of their recent-onset psychotic patients killed themselves over the 4 years that the patients were followed up. Although prediction can never be absolute, younger male patients appear at particular risk, as are those of high IQ who previously showed good social and occupational functioning. Dysphoric or depressive symptoms, a past history of attempted suicide and drug or alcohol abuse are also useful predictors.[35]

Violence

Violent behaviour by the psychotic patient is to be avoided at all costs, as even its threat can permanently alter the patient's life, for example by leading to referral to a high-security forensic establishment. Serious violence tends to be perpetrated by patients at a later stage of their illness and the main predictors are similar to those for violence in the general population: male sex, unemployment and drug and alcohol abuse. Of course, a diagnosis of schizophrenia or paranoid illness increases risk.[36]

Before the onset of frank psychosis

3

It has become clear in recent years that, in many cases, the onset of psychosis does not come out of the blue but rather is the culmination of a trajectory of increasing deviance. This chapter will therefore discuss

1. the childhood antecedents of psychosis
2. the prodromal phase and
3. risk factors

Childhood antecedents

A number of approaches have been adopted to establish the childhood function of those who later become psychotic.

Retrospective studies

Researchers have interviewed the mothers of psychotic patients and asked them retrospectively about their child's development. For example, Foerster *et al* noted that mothers recalled their preschizophrenic children as having shown developmental problems particularly with reading, and an excess of schizoid and schizotypal traits.[37,38] Similarly, Cannon *et al* collected data on childhood function from the mothers of 70 schizophrenic and 28 bipolar patients.[39] Both groups showed poorer adjustment in childhood than controls; however, the preschizophrenics were five times more likely to fall into the worst adjustment group than the bipolar patients.

Follow-back studies

Researchers have gone back to the clinical records of those adult psychotic patients who were seen earlier by child psychiatrists. Preschizophrenic children may show low IQ and poor scholastic performance.

Videotape studies

A particularly novel approach was employed by Walker and her colleagues[40]; they obtained videotapes of children who subsequently became schizophrenic and 'blindly' compared the videos with those of their growing siblings. The preschizophrenics were more likely to show motor abnormalities such as clumsiness or odd movements.

Cohort studies

A fourth approach avoids the biases intrinsic to all the above studies by following up unselected samples of children into adult life. Thus, Jones *et al* examined the life histories of 4746 children who had been born 1 week in 1946 in the UK, and who had been examined many times by the age of 43 years.[41] The 30 children who went on to develop schizophrenia had slightly delayed motor milestones (eg walking). At ages 4 and 6, the preschizophrenic children were more likely to play alone than the normal children, and by age 8 they already performed more poorly on cognitive tests. Interestingly, as in the videotape study discussed above, they were more likely to show abnormal motor movements. Thus, not all the abnormal movements shown by schizophrenic patients can be ascribed to antipsychotic medication!

It is clear that a proportion of schizophrenics show deficits in motor, cognitive and social performance long before they develop psychotic symptoms. What is not clear is

1. whether or not there exists a distinct subgroup only which is typified by childhood abnormality or
2. whether the childhood deficits are an early intrinsic manifestation of the schizophrenic process or whether such abnormalities are simply risk factors for the later onset of the schizophrenia syndrome[41,42]

Furthermore, the specificity of this finding remains in doubt, as evidence has emerged suggesting that some individuals with affective disorder and nonschizophrenic psychosis show neurological abnormalities and subtle differences in social and cognitive development, similar to those found in patients with schizophrenia.[43] For example, in the same prospective study of a national birth cohort as examined by Jones *et al*,[41] Van Os and colleagues[22] showed that delay in achieving milestones, speech defects and poorer cognitive performance were also associated with increased risk of chronic depression. The main difference was that the childhood

dysfunction of the predepressives tended to be less severe than that of the preschizophrenics, and they were more likely to have been regarded as 'gloomy' by their school doctor at age 7.

Children of psychotic parents

Researchers have studied the children of psychotic parents. The best known of these 'high-risk' studies is that of Parnas et al in Denmark.[44] These authors chose 200 pre-adolescent and teenage offspring of schizophrenic mothers and matched them with 100 low-risk children; the average age of both groups was 15 years and they were followed up for 6 years. By that time 20 of the high-risk children had had a psychiatric breakdown; this 'sick' group were distinguished particularly by a history of birth and pregnancy complications and on the original testing had shown more deviant autonomic responsivity. A second study by Mednick *et al*[45] found lowered birth weights in high-risk children while Schulsinger *et al*[46] demonstrated that it is particularly those offspring who have suffered obstetric complications who develop schizophrenia.

Prepsychotic or prodromal phase

Before frank psychosis emerges, patients may experience *prodromal symptoms*. Keith and Matthews described the prodrome as a heterogeneous group of behaviours temporally related to the onset of psychosis.[47] Loebel *et al* defined it as the time interval from onset of unusual behavioural symptoms to onset of psychotic symptoms,[5] while Beiser *et al* interpreted the term as meaning the period from first noticeable symptoms to onset of actual psychotic symptoms.[7]

The prodrome appears to combine generic stress responses, such as dysphoric mood states, sleep disturbance and social withdrawal, with the early features of the psychotic episode, such as perceptual and information process-ing defects (Table 3). Such symptoms are nonspecific, not uncommon in adolescence and, by definition, are pre-rather than psychotic. Furthermore, since the concept of prodrome is essen-tially a retrospective one, the accuracy of recall is an issue. Recall may be affected by a long delay between initial changes and the development of obvious psychotic symptoms.[48] It may also be altered by 'effort after meaning', that is patients or their families search for something that appeared to be associ-

Table 3
Prodromal features most commonly described in first-episode psychosis.

• *Changes in mood: depression, anxiety, mood swings, irritability*
• *Changes in cognition: odd or unusual ideas, vagueness, deterioration in study or work*
• *Changes in perception of self and the world*
• *Changed behaviours, eg withdrawal and loss of interest in socializing, suspiciousness, deterioration in role functioning*
• *Physical changes: in sleep and appetite, loss of energy, reduced drive and motivation*
From Yung and McGorry[51]

ated with the beginning of all the changes and date their stories from that time.[49,50] The mental state of the patient at the time when the history is taken is also likely to influence the light in which it is told. Finally, some families feel enormous guilt and responsibility for failing to have noticed a problem in the early stages and this can also affect their memory of the timing of the first symptoms.

An alternative approach as proposed by Yung and McGorry is to consider such prodromal periods as those of 'at risk mental state'.[51] This ensures that there is the possibility that not all such 'at risk' periods inevitably progress to the development of frank psychosis. It also allows for any one individual potentially to experience a number of such episodes of 'at risk mental state' and on occasion to recover from these, depending on the interplay of various other factors known to increase the probability of a psychotic episode (such as life events, family stress). The designation of specific criteria to identify such an at risk state might include:

• a definite change in social functioning from a baseline level
• the presence of particular symptomatology such as change in perception, ideas of reference or delusional mood or
• schizotypal personality disorder[19]

The prodrome may proceed to psychosis, but some patients progress no further and regain their normal equanimity. However, it is important to remember that, as yet, there are no data available on the relative risk of transition from such prodromal symptoms to an episode of frank psychosis. Is it therefore appropriate to intervene in such cases as if a definite diagnosis of psychosis had already been made? There are a number of compli-

cated ethical issues involved in the treatment of these patients, as there is likely to be a significant number of false positives detected in any given sample of adolescents or young adults. It is likely that such cases would remit without specific treatment, and it could be argued that the risk of treating them is not justified.

The existence of childhood characteristics and prodromal symptoms which are statistically associated with the development of psychosis has led to questions of whether large programmes to identify such individuals should be established. Van Os *et al*[31] have advised caution on the basis that:

1. the known risk factors are only weak predictors
2. therefore, most individuals so identified would not become psychotic
3. intervention might not be effective, and certainly would not be cost-effective

However, Yung *et al* have suggested that it may be possible to identify adolescents who have a high likelihood (approaching 50%) of developing a psychotic episode.[52] This group use not only symptoms and signs to identify this group, but also traits such as family history of psychosis and also the fact that the individuals were part of a sample which had already been referred to an early psychosis unit as possible psychotics.

Risk factors

A number of factors are associated with an increased *risk* of psychosis, some of which appear causal. Much evidence suggests that there is considerable overlap in the risk factors which operate across the range of psychoses, and that biological risk factors are more frequently identified in early-onset than late-onset cases.

The risk factors for first-episode psychoses may be usefully broken down into:

- *predisposing factors*
  genetic
  early environmental hazards
- *precipitating factors*
  adverse life events
  drug abuse

Predisposing factors

Genetic

Family studies
Psychotic disorders cluster in families, that is the relatives of an affected

person also have an increased risk of developing a psychotic disorder;[53] this is particularly so where the affected person had an early onset of illness. Thus, the relatives of patients with early-onset schizophrenia[54] and early onset affective disorder[55] have a higher risk of a related condition than the relatives of late-onset cases.

There is also a tendency for the different psychoses to 'breed true', but this is not an absolute rule. Several family studies have found that the relatives of individuals with schizophrenia are at increased risk not only of schizophrenia but also of other psychoses and related personality disorders;[56] similarly, the children of parents with bipolar affective disorder have an increased risk of schizophrenia. Furthermore, studies of families with several psychotic members show that schizophrenia and affective disorder can occur in the same family, while the relatives of patients with schizoaffective disorder are known to have an increased risk of both schizophrenia and affective psychoses.[57] Owing to the guilt which many families feel with the onset of psychosis in a family member, it may be very difficult to elicit an accurate family history, especially where more subtle disturbances exist in other family members.

Twin studies

A twin pair is said to be congruent if both members of the pair are affected, discordant if only one is affected. A genetic effect is indicated if the monozygotic (MZ) concordance rate is significantly greater than the dizygotic (DZ). Twin studies for schizophrenia show MZ concordance rates of 31–58%, DZ concordance rates of 4–27%[53]; for bipolar affective disorder the MZ concordance is even higher, at 79%, with the DZ concordance rate being 19%.[58]

Adoption studies

In schizophrenia, all adoption studies to date are consistent with a significant genetic contribution to the disorder.[59,60,61,62] There are fewer adoption studies in bipolar affective disorder; however, Mendlewicz and Rainer showed that 28% of the biological parents of bipolar adoptees had affective illness (mainly unipolar) compared with 12% of their adopting parents.[63]

Linkage studies

In linkage analysis the degree of linkage of genetic markers of known chromosomal location is analysed with respect to the psychiatric condition, ie the degree of cosegregation of genetic markers with the disorder is investigated. Linkage studies in schizophrenia have produced conflicting results[64] as have those in bipolar[65].

Association studies

In this approach particular genes implicated through other means as being involved in psychosis are selected, and a search is made for differences in distribution of the alleles of the gene between patients and controls. If found, such differences suggest that this gene influences susceptibility to psychosis or lies in close approximation to a disease gene. Candidate genes tested in psychosis include those involved in dopaminergic and serotonergic pathways, immune processing and neurodevelopment. In schizophrenia, positive (but also negative) associations have been reported for allelic variants of the dopamine D_3 receptor,[66,67] the $5HT_{2A}$ receptor[68] and at the highly polymorphic HLA locus.[68,69] In bipolar affective disorder, a functional variation in the promotor region of the serotonin transporter gene has been associated with the disorder.[70]

Association studies may also use genetic markers (rather than known genes).[71]

Increasing severity and earlier age of onset of psychosis in successive generations have been observed in some families. This has led to suggestions that 'anticipation' may be operating. 'Anticipation' occurs in a number of neurological disorders, and is known to arise from the expansion of trinucleotide repeats between generations.[72] Researchers have therefore screened psychotic patients for such trinucleotide repeats. A significant shift towards larger repeat sizes has been reported in those affected with schizophrenia or bipolar affective disorder,[73,74] but other studies have been negative. One possibility is that such repeat expansions may be found particularly in those psychotic patients who have very early (ie childhood) onset and in whom genetic factors are thought to play a particularly significant role.

Early environmental hazards

The combined effect of the putative genetic factors in bipolar affective disorder and in schizoaffective disorder is very much greater than that of the environment. The genetic effect also seems to be stronger for these two conditions than for schizophrenia. Cannon and Jones have analysed in

detail the relative importance of various risk factors for schizophrenia (Table 4).[75] Paradoxically, we know very little about which specific genes are involved and more regarding the specific environmental factors implicated.

Intrauterine and perinatal

Obstetric complications have been repeatedly shown to be a risk factor for developing schizophrenia.[76,77] The early findings were criticised on the grounds that many studies relied upon maternal recall of the history of pre- and perinatal events. However, studies that examined original birth records have also consistently reported more obstetric complications in schizophrenia than in controls.[78–80] Obstetric complications have been reported in particular among patients with an early onset.[81]

The obstetric complications implicated have included:

* low birth weight
* prematurity and 'small for dates' status
* pre-eclampsia
* prolonged labour and
* asphyxia

Most of the studies on which these claims have been made were rather

Table 4
'Best-estimates' of effect sizes of various genetic and environmental risk factors for schizophrenia (expressed as odds ratios or relative risks).[75]

Category of risk factor	Specific risk factor	Best estimate of effect size
Genetic	MZ twin of schizophrenic patient	46
	DZ twin of schizophrenic patient	14
	Child/sibling of schizophrenic patient	10
Pre- and perinatal environment	Birth complications	2
	Severe undernutrition (1st trimester)	2
	Maternal influenza (2nd trimester)	2
	'Unwanted pregnancy'	2
Developmental	Delayed milestones	3
	Speech problems	3
Postnatal	Chronic cannabis consumption	2

small but a recent meta-analysis of data pooled from 854 schizophrenic patients and controls has confirmed these claims, and suggests that the common factor be risk of hypoxic-ischaemic brain damage. It has also been shown that schizophrenic patients have a lower birthweight than the general population.[81] Preschizophrenics also tend to have a smaller head circumference at birth than controls,[78,80,83] implicating earlier impairment of brain growth.

Prenatal exposure to viral infection has been implicated. Patients with schizophrenia and bipolar disorder show a slight excess of winter–spring births and a deficit in births in late summer and autumn.[84,85] Various theories have been put forward to explain this association, the most widely debated postulating prenatal exposure to winter-borne viral infection with resulting subtle brain damage. The fact that the winter/spring excess is greatest for those born in cities suggests an infection whose spread is facilitated by winter and by crowding, and has therefore focused attention on influenza epidemics which show such a pattern. Isohanni et al have shown associations between maternal fever and schizophrenia and also between childhood cerebral infection or convulsions and later schizophrenia.[86]

Brain structure

Numerous studies using CT and MRI have shown subtle abnormalities of brain structure in schizophrenia. Lateral and third ventricular enlargement are the most consistent neuroanatomical changes found, but MRI studies also show an increase in sulcal size and CSF space in general.[87] The increase in fluid space is likely to be due to a decrease in brain volume. Indeed, recent MRI reports suggest generalized cortical grey matter volume decrements in schizophrenia of the order of 5–10%.[88,89] Postmortem studies have largely confirmed the neuroimaging findings.[90,91]

Neuroimaging studies during the *first* episode of schizophrenia show abnormalities, and studies following up patients for up to 8 years in general do not show a progression of the abnormalities. These findings, and the evidence that the abnormalities tend to

be worse in patients with an *early* onset of psychosis, suggest that the abnormalities are secondary to an impairment in the process of neurodevelopment.

A neurodevelopmental hypothesis has been proposed which states that a substantial group of schizophrenic patients have experienced a disturbance of the orderly development of the brain, decades before the symptomatic phase of the illness begins.[92,93]

Gene–environment interaction

It seems to be the *interaction* between genetic and environmental effects which is crucial for the genesis of psychosis: an interaction between rearing and biological vulnerability has also been reported.[62,94] Obstetric complications may also interact with genetic factors to increase the risk of schizophrenia.[95–97]

As shown in Figure 1, there may be an underlying vulnerability to psychotic disorders which is normally distributed in the population, and determined by a combination of genetic (polygenic) and environmental effects, with only those whose vulnerability exceeds a threshold manifesting psychosis. An additional environmental factor acting on subgroup of the population could shift the curve towards the threshold.

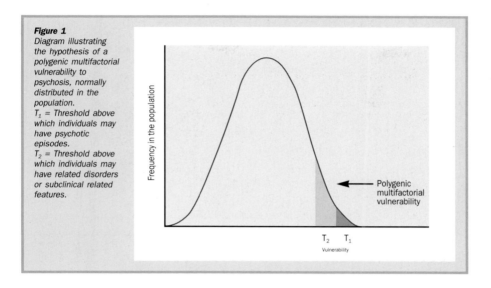

Figure 1
Diagram illustrating the hypothesis of a polygenic multifactorial vulnerability to psychosis, normally distributed in the population.
T_1 = Threshold above which individuals may have psychotic episodes.
T_2 = Threshold above which individuals may have related disorders or subclinical related features.

Precipitating factors

As discussed in the previous section, distant predisposing factors, either genetic factors or early developmental damage, predispose individuals to psychotic breakdown. However, they do not explain why individuals break down at a particular time point. In the context of first-episode psychosis, precipitating factors occurring near the actual onset are of obvious interest, particularly since such factors may be more open to therapeutic intervention than genetic or other biological predisposition. Certainly, patients often suffer their first breakdown following the operation of obvious precipitating factors. The two most obvious are adverse life events and drug abuse.

Life events

Stress can precipitate psychotic illness. There is general agreement that adverse life events play an important aetiological role in affective disorder.[98] An excess of stressful life events in the 3 weeks before the onset (or relapse) of schizophrenic illness has been reported.[99] More recently, support for an association between life events and onset of psychosis has come from three studies which introduced important methodological improvements.[100–102] However, most authorities regard social adversity as operating on already predisposed individuals, not as primary causal factors in their own right. Thus it has been suggested that life events serve to trigger the onset of symptoms in those who are predisposed and are experiencing tense and difficult situations.[103]

Drug abuse

Clinicians commonly consider that psychosis can be precipitated by drug abuse, and an association between drug consumption and onset of psychosis has often been reported. However, it is often difficult to exclude the possibility that the drugs were being taken in a vain attempt to self medicate already existing psychopathology.[104] Psychotic symptoms often arise following abuse of drugs, particularly

- dopamine agonists such as amphetamine and cocaine

- hallucinogenic drugs such as LSD, PCP and ecstasy and
- cannabis

There is not much doubt about the role of the first two classes. For instance, amphetamine- or PCP-induced psychoses can mimic many of the symptoms of schizophrenia. Outside the USA, amphetamine psychosis is more frequently observed, generally in those who have consumed enormous quantities of the drug over prolonged periods. It usually resolves within a few days of ceasing the abuse.

However, the role of cannabis is hotly disputed. The psychoses associated with it seem to be more polymorphic with both schizophrenic or affective symptoms.[105] There is some limited evidence that cannabis consumption is associated with an increased risk[106] and a poor outcome or increased relapse rate of psychosis.[107,108] It has been shown that the relatives of psychotic probands with a positive urine test for cannabis had a significantly higher morbid risk of schizophrenia than did relatives of probands with a negative urine test.[102] One possible interpretation is that cannabis consumption may precipitate psychosis in those carrying some susceptibility gene(s); an alternative is that one cannabis consuming sibling passed on the habit of heavy abuse to another.

There is no clear evidence concerning whether abuse of any drug can cause life-long schizophrenia or affective disorder, *de novo*. Most expert opinion suggests that, as with adverse life events, some pre-existing biological vulnerability is necessary. However, such beliefs tend to an article of faith since there is little data on which to base them.

Schizophrenia versus affective psychosis

There is little evidence for a particular causal factor being specific to a diagnostic category within the functional psychoses. Rather, the evidence indicates quantitative, but not qualitative differences between the categories of schizophrenia and affective psychosis. Familial morbid risk of schizophrenia and neurodevelopmental factors (eg obstetric complications, decreased brain volume) operate preferentially, though not specifically, at the end of the psychopathological spectrum characterised by insidious onset and a preponderance of negative features. Familial morbid risk of affective disorder and adverse life events act at the end associated with acute onset, a predominance of affective features and a dearth of negative symptoms.

Antipsychotics: pharmacology

4

Therapeutic and side-effects

The first drug to be prescribed for the treatment of psychosis was chlorpromazine.[110] Over the ensuing 35 years, many other drugs of similar pharmacological profile followed; these are termed 'conventional' or 'typical' antipsychotics. However, in the early 1990s the situation changed with the marketing of clozapine in most Western nations as the first antipsychotic with a significantly different profile, both in animal and human studies. It was termed an 'atypical' antipsychotic, on the basis of a lower potential to induce extrapyramidal side-effects.[111] Since then other, similar antipsychotics have been synthesized, and although there is some difference of opinion as to what constitutes the definition of an atypical antipsychotic, it is generally agreed that they fulfil the criteria given in Table 5.[112]

Table 5
Properties of atypical antipsychotics (from Lieberman[112]).

Properties of atypical antipsychotic drugs

*Superior antipsychotic efficacy in some measure
eg in refractory patients, or against negative
symptoms and/or cognitive deficits
Produce lower levels of EPS including tardive
dyskinesia*

Conventional antipsychotics

There are four categories of conventional antipsychotics:

• phenothiazines (with three different subtypes)

• butyrophenones
• thioxanthines
• diphenylbutylpiperidines

Examples of each are given in Table 6.

At clinical doses, all conventional antipsychotics have an affinity for the dopamine D_2 receptor, plus a varying spectrum of affinities for other neuroreceptors. For example, chlorpromazine was marketed by the French pharmaceutical company Rhône-Poulenc as '*largactyl*' owing to its *large* range of *act*ions, reflecting its broad spectrum of affinities.

Conventional antipsychotics differ in their propensity to induce sedation, anticholinergic (antimuscarinic) and extrapyramidal side-effects (EPS).[113] The differences between the three phenothiazine groups are shown in Table 7.

Table 6
Conventional antipsychotics.

	Chemical group	Drugs
1a	Phenothiazine (aliphatic)	Chlorpromazine, promazine
1b	Phenothiazine (piperidine)	Thioridazine
1c	Phenothiazine (piperazine)	Trifluoperazine, fluphenazine
2	Butyrophenone	Haloperidol, droperidol
3	Thioxanthines	Flupenthixol, zuclopenthixol
4	Diphenylbutylpiperidine	Pimozide

Table 7
Properties of phenothiazines.

Chemical group	Sedation	Antimuscarinic	EPS
Phenothiazine (aliphatic)	+++	++	++
Phenothiazine (piperidine)	++	+++	+
Phenothiazine (piperazine)	+	+	+++

Conventional antipsychotics of other chemical groups tend to resemble the piperazine phenothiazines. These differential effects can be understood in terms of their differential affinities[114] for:

- the histamine H_1 receptor (sedation): chlorpromazine>thioridazine> fluphenazine
- the muscarinic m1 receptor (antimuscarinic effects): thioridazine>chlorpromazine> haloperidol
- the m1/D_2 ratio (amelioration of EPS): thioridazine>chlorpromazine> fluphenazine

An attractively simple rule is that low-potency high milligram compounds (eg chlorpromazine, thioridazine) are associated with higher rates of sedation and anticholinergic effects, but lower rates of EPS. On the other hand, high-potency low milligram drugs (eg haloperidol, pimozide) are less sedative and less anticholinergic, but have higher rates of EPS.

For most typical antipsychotics elimination is principally hepatic, undergoing metabolism by the hepatic cytochrome P450 system, including the polymorphic CYP2D6; drug interactions at this site are discussed in a later section.

Atypical or new antipsychotics

The atypical antipsychotics introduced in the 1990s may be divided into two groups: those which are structurally similar to clozapine (including olanzapine and quetiapine) and those which are structurally distinct from clozapine and each other but similar to each other in their receptor profiles (risperidone, sertindole and ziprasidone).[114]

Clozapine has a broad spectrum of receptor affinities. It has a high affinity for serotonin receptors (notably 5-HT_{2A}, 5-HT_6 and 5-HT_{2C}, and to a lesser extent, 5-HT_3), with clinically relevant affinities also for the α_1-adrenergic, the m1-muscarinic, the H_1-histaminergic and α_2-adrenergic receptors.[114,115] It also has a high affinity for the dopamine D_4 receptor, with only moderate affinities for the D_2, D_1 and D_3 receptors. Olanzapine has a similar profile to clozapine in in vitro receptor binding, but has a higher affinity for the D_1 and D_2 receptors.

The second group of drugs are all similar in having a high affinity for, and antagonism at, dopamine D_2 and serotonin 5-HT_2-receptors, and are known as serotonin-dopamine antagonists (SDAs).[115] They also show significant affinity for the α_1-adrenoreceptor, with sertindole and ziprasidone having a higher affinity than risperidone for the D_1 receptor.

To some extent the rule regarding potency and side-effects for typicals given above holds for atypicals: clozapine is a low-potency, high milligram compound which has significant sedative and anticholinergic effects but little or no EPS. Risperidone is a high-potency, low

milligram drug which has few sedative and anticholinergic effects and at doses of less than 4 mg leads to a reduction in baseline levels of EPS in drug-naive first episode cases.[116] However, olanzapine breaks the rule in that it is used in low milligram dosage but has a significant sedative and anticholinergic effect.

The atypical antipsychotics are metabolized by polymorphic cytochromes (especially CYP1A2, CYP2D6 and CYP3A); their clearance is therefore subject to variables affecting the activity of these cytochromes, such as age, cigarette smoking and drug interactions. Olanzapine is also metabolized significantly by N-glucuronidation (a phase II oxidative process not involving the CYP system) and by the flavin–monooxygenase system, which means that its metabolism is less dependent on the polymorphic and inducible cytochrome systems.

Understanding the receptor profiles

Knowledge of the range of effects elicited by blockade of specific neuroreceptors (Table 8) helps to elucidate both the therapeutic and side-effects generated by a given antipsychotic. The higher the in vivo occupancy by a drug

Table 8
Correlations between receptor blockade and adverse effects.

Receptor type	Adverse effects
Dopamine (D_2)	EPS, sexual dysfunction secondary to prolactin elevation
Muscarinic (esp m1)	Blurred vision, dry mouth, constipation, difficulty with micturition, precipitation or exacerbation of glaucoma, sinus tachycardia and QRS changes, dysmnesia, acute confusional state
Histamine (esp H_1)	Sedation, weight gain
Serotonin	Increased appetite, possible contribution to sedation, hypotension and ejaculatory problems
Adrenergic	Orthostatic hypotension, nasal congestion, delayed ejaculation

in its clinical dose range for a specific receptor, the more likely it is to elicit the clinical effects resulting from blockade of that specific receptor type, unless there is a mitigating influence from blockade of another receptor.

Affinity data may predict in vivo occupancies, although the correlation is not absolute. Furthermore, a drug with a relatively low affinity for a receptor can achieve the same degree of receptor blockade as a drug of relatively high affinity if, due to the administration of a higher dose, the lower affinity drug is present at a higher concentration at the receptor site. It should also be noted that if the dose is increased to gain increased blockade of a particular receptor (eg D_2), then other receptors may also be affected, with consequent side effects.

Therapeutic effects

Against the positive psychotic symptoms

There are several longstanding hypotheses regarding the effect of antipsychotics on positive psychotic symptoms, based on the blockade of dopamine and serotonin receptors.

Dopamine receptors

Seeman and colleagues provided convincing evidence for the role of the D_2 receptor by showing a linear correlation between the average daily clinical dose of various typical antipsychotics and their potency in displacement of [3H]-haloperidol from D_2 receptor binding sites in vitro.[117] The hypothesis that the higher the D_2 blockade, the greater the antipsychotic effect, was largely accepted until the early 1990s when neuroimaging data showed that clozapine had a lower occupancy of D_2 sites despite a greater antipsychotic efficacy than typical antipsychotics in patients with refractory schizophrenia.[118,119]

Attention switched to the dopamine D_4 receptor with the claim by Van Tol's group that clozapine's antipsychotic effect was via D_4,[120] but this finding was subsequently disputed.[121] In a recent neuroimaging study, a three-fold elevation of 'D_4-like' sites was found in schizophrenia,[122] but again this was disputed. D_1 receptors have also been implicated in the effects of antipsychotics on negative symptoms,[123] and there have been reports of association between allelic variation in D_3 and treatment response as well as with schizophrenia itself.[66,67,124,125]

There has been a renaissance of interest in D_2, with the in vivo demonstration that although clozapine exerts lower striatal D_2 blockade, it is associated with limbic D_2 blockade equal to that of typical antipsychotics.[126,127] The relevance of this is that much research implicates the temporal lobe in the generation of positive psychotic symptoms.[128,129]

Serotonin receptors

Serotonergic theories of schizophrenia stretch back to the evidence that many hallucinogens, and possibly endogenous hallucinogens,[130] act on serotonin receptors. The front-runner in the search for those receptors implicated in antipsychotic effects has been the 5-HT_{2A} receptor. Possession of the T102C allelic variant of this receptor has been associated with poor response to clozapine,[131] and with schizophrenia itself,[68] although the results in various studies are conflicting. The 5-HT_{2C} receptor co-localizes with the 5-HT_{2A} in the medial prefrontal cortex, and a variant of the 5-HT_{2C} may also influence response to clozapine.[132,133]

Other receptors

Hypotheses concerning the action of antipsychotics have been put forward implicating glutamate, noradrenaline, sigma opioid, GABA, glycine, indeed, almost every conceivably relevant receptor system. The sigma opioid receptor has been a particular favourite since some typical and atypical antipsychotics show a substantial affinity for it; a role for sigma ligands in the modulation of dopaminergic and glutamatergic transmissions has been postulated.

Against the negative symptoms of schizophrenia

Again, there are several hypotheses regarding the neurotransmitter mechanisms responsible for the generation of negative symptoms, and hence for the pharmacological alleviation of these. One theory is based on hypodopaminergic function (D_1) in the prefrontal cortex, which might be antagonized by blockade of 5-HT$_{2A}$ receptors. In support of this are the results of a trial using ritanserin (a selective 5-HT$_{2A}$ and 5-HT$_{2C}$ antagonist), showing an apparent reduction in negative symptoms.[135]

Another suggestion involves the modulation of dopaminergic transmission by sigma receptor blockade; a selective sigma antagonist has been claimed to show a beneficial effect on the negative symptoms of schizophrenia.[136]

Side-effects

Extrapyramidal symptoms

It is widely accepted that reduced dopaminergic function in the nigrostriatal pathway leads to parkinsonism and other EPS. Blockade of the 5-HT$_{2A}$ receptors on the substantia nigra DA cells increases dopaminergic neurotransmission; hence 5-HT$_{2A}$ antagonism lessens the reduction in dopaminergic function caused by blockade of D_2 receptors.[137] All the new antipsychotics, except quetiapine, have a higher affinity for 5-HT$_{2A}$ receptors than for D_2 (a 5-HT$_{2A}$/D_2 ratio grater than 1); this is thought to explain at least part of their lower propensity to induce EPS. The rank order for the 5-HT$_{2A}$/D_2 ratio (calculated from the molar equilibrium dissociations)[114] is:

> clozapine>chlorpromazine>
> risperidone>olanzapine>
> thioridazine>sertindole>
> quetiapine>haloperidol>fluphenazine

There is also an inverse relationship between the affinity of antipsychotics for muscarinic receptors and their propensity to induce EPS,[114] which holds true for both the conventional and new antipsychotics. There are five subtypes of muscarinic receptor, the m1 being the most abundant and the m5 the least abundant in most areas of the human brain. Olanzapine and clozapine have high affinity and selectivity for the m1 receptor; the affinity of thioridazine for the m1 receptor is in between that of olanzapine and clozapine:[114,138]

olanzapine>thioridazine>clozapine>
chlorpromazine>quetiapine>
haloperidol>risperidone

Risperidone is the only antipsychotic with no anticholinergic activity,[138] which is a positive point – as this means it does not have the anticholinergic side effects including cognitive impairment. As mentioned above, antipsychotics which appear to exert a lower striatal D_2 than limbic D_2 blockade (clozapine and quetiapine[126,139]) may have a relatively low likelihood of inducing EPS. In clinical trials (not specifically first episode) of olanzapine, sertindole, quetiapine, and less than 10 mg of risperidone, the incidence of EPS is similar to that on placebo.[139–142] This does not, of course, imply a zero incidence of EPS; many patients on placebo will have recordable EPS owing either to their spontaneous occurrence or to prior treatment with typical antipsychotics. For first episode patients a dose as low as possible should be prescribed.

Tardive dyskinesia

As TD is a complication of the chronic use of antipsychotics, one might think it unimportant in the care of patients with a first episode of psychosis. However,

since many first-episode patients will continue to be prescribed antipsychotics in the long term, it is important that they receive drugs which carry the minimum risk of TD.

Recent evidence suggests that agents which are associated with a low incidence of EPS may also have a low risk of inducing TD. Evidence in support of this comes from

1. a prospective study of elderly patients receiving antipsychotics which showed that those with EPS had a significantly greater likelihood of developing TD[143]
2. a larger prospective study over 45 years of 226 patients who received antipsychotics and in whom tremor was noted as a risk factor for TD[144]

Critics point out that movements clinically indistinguishable from TD are seen in 5–15% of elderly individuals who have never received antipsychotic drugs.[145] None the less, it does appear that agents, such as clozapine, associated with a low incidence of EPS, are also associated with a low incidence of TD; indeed, clozapine is used to *treat* TD. The overall annual incidence for new instances of TD with risperidone by June 1997 was 0.0006%, significantly lower than that reported with typical neuroleptics (3–6%).[146]

The pharmacodynamic basis of tardive dyskinesia has not been established. Animal studies and some clinical studies with D_1 selective antagonists indicate that D_1 antagonism may be protective against TD.[147] A recent report indicates that individuals homozygous for an allelic variant of the dopamine D_3 receptor gene may have an increased risk of developing TD.[148]

Sedation

There are three types of histamine receptor: H_1 is involved in arousal and the regulation of appetite, H_2 with gastric secretion and H_3 has a neuromodulatory effect. Many antipsychotics are more potent than the classic antihistamine diphenhydramine at blocking histamine H_1 receptors; rank order of H_1 affinity is:[114]

clozapine>olanzapine> chlorpromazine>quetiapine> diphenhydramine>thioridazine> fluphenazine>risperidone> sertindole>haloperidol

Cholinergic effects

The effects of muscarinic blockade (principally m1) are given in Table 8. Cognitive deficits more subtle than those shown in Table 8 may also be attributable to muscarinic blockade. The lack of muscarinic blockade may explain risperidone effect in improving cognitive deficit in schizophrenia.[149] Interestingly, clozapine appears to have muscarinic agonist as well as antagonist activity, the agonism occurring at the m4 receptor.[150] The drooling of saliva (sialorrhoea) produced by clozapine can be at least partially relieved by a muscarinic antagonist such as pirenzepine.[151,152]

Weight gain

Weight gain may be mediated by H_1 or serotonin antagonism, or both. Chlorpromazine has a high H_1 and 5-HT_{2A} affinity; the majority of patients receiving chlorpromazine when it was first introduced gained considerable amounts of weight. Clozapine is associated with weight gain in an average of 50% of cases, and other atypical drugs with high H_1 affinity such as olanzapine share this effect. Risperidone and ziprasidone appear to have a lower tendency to induce weight gain.

Sexual dysfunction

The tuberoinfundibular DA pathway mediates inhibition of the release of prolactin from the anterior pituitary via D$_2$ receptors; blockade of this effect therefore leads to an increase in prolactin levels, which can result in oligomenorrhoea and galactorrhoea in women and reduced sexual function and gynaecomastia in men. Sexual dysfunction is a known effect of a number of antipsychotics.

Pharmacokinetics

A lack of knowledge of the pharmacokinetics of antipsychotic drugs can result in the first-episode patient being exposed to inappropriate doses of medication with resultant impaired efficacy or unpleasant side-effects; such an event can permanently impair the patient's trust in the psychiatric services. The correct application of pharmacokinetic principles can, therefore, make a major contribution to the more effective use of pharmacotherapy in the care of first-episode patients. For example, owing to the large interindividual variability (on average 30-fold differences in blood level result from the same dosage of a medication administered to a population[141]) most antipsychotics require individual dosage titration according to the clinical response.

Absorption

Food consumption does not significantly affect the absorption of most typical and atypical antipsychotics, but does increase that of quetiapine and ziprasidone.[153] A slow release oral formulation has been developed for quetiapine. The comparative pharmacokinetics of the atypicals is given in Table 9.

In situations in which a rapid effect is desirable, IM (eg droperidol or haloperidol) or oral liquid formulation (eg chlorpromazine) may be indicated. For very rapid tranquilization, IV antipsychotics and/or IV benzodiazepines may be used.[154] The formulation for depot preparations gives an absorption rate that is slow enough to be the main determinant of the time for the drug to reach steady state.

Distribution

Most antipsychotics are very lipid soluble and protein bound, and therefore move rapidly from blood to tissue. The free drug concentration is affected by factors which influence the amount of available plasma protein for drug binding. Factors such as malnutrition or liver disease which reduce the available

Table 9
Comparative pharmacokinetics of oral doses of the atypical antipsychotics.[141]

Drug	$T_{max}(h)$*	Mean $t_{1/2}(h)$†	Steady state (days)‡	Effect of food
Risperidone	1	3.5		No change
9-OH-risperidone	3	22	4–6	
Clozapine	3	16	4–8	No change
Olanzapine	5	30	5–7	No change
Sertindole	10	55–90§	7–14	No change
Quetiapine	1¶	7	1–2	Increases
Ziprasidone	5	4–10‖	1–3	Increases

*$T_{max}(h)$ is the time in hours from dose administration to when the maximum plasma concentration is attained.
†$t_{1/2}(h)$ is the half-life in hours.
‡The equilibrium state in which the amount of drug administered is counterbalanced by the amount of drug eliminated.
§Variation due to CYP2D6 polymorphism.
¶For quetiapine SR, T_{max} is 5 h.
‖Dose dependent.

plasma protein increase the free drug concentration and vice versa.

Elimination

The rate of elimination determines the half-life. Drugs with a half-life approximating to 24 hours may be administered once daily; this applies in most cases to risperidone, and to olanzapine and sertindole. In commencing medica-

tion for a patient with his/her first episode of psychosis, it is important to know when a steady state will be achieved. A pharmacokinetic rule is that at least 90% of the steady-state level is reached within four times the half-life of any drug; in five times the half-life >98% of the steady state concentration is attained.

The major pathways of elimination for the currently prescribable atypical antipsychotics are given in Table 10.

Table 10
Elimination pathways for atypical antipsychotics.[153]

Drug	CYP1A2	CYP2D6	CYP3A	Other
Risperidone		++		Conjugation plus renal excretion for 9-OH-risperidone
Clozapine	++	+	+	CYP2E1, FMO
Olanzapine	++	+		FMO, glucuronidation
Sertindole		++	++	Faecal excretion

CYP: cytochrome P450.

The cytochromes

Phase I hepatic metabolism is conducted largely by a polymorphic superfamily of enzymes, the cytochrome P450s (CYPs).[155] Of these, four have been identified as being important in the metabolism of antipsychotics: CYP1A2, CYP2C19, CYP2D6 and CYP3A4.

It is important to understand the role of these cytochromes in the metabolism of antipsychotics because:

- they are polymorphic, ie there is significant inter-individual variation in activity
- CYP1A2 and CYP3A4 are inducible
- drug–drug interactions take place at the level of these cytochromes

Thus it is possible to predict whether or not two drugs are likely to interact with each other at the CYP level by knowing:

- which CYP(s) is/are mainly responsible for the metabolism of the drugs
- the relative contribution of the CYP(s) to the total metabolism of the drugs
- the relative affinities of the drugs for the CYP(s)
- the relative concentrations of the drugs in hepatocytes as judged from plasma concentrations

If two drugs are metabolized by the same CYP, a competitive inhibition can be predicted, and the metabolism of the drug with least affinity for the enzyme may be inhibited.[156]

CYP2D6

CYP2D6 plays a central role in the metabolism of many typical antipsy-

Table 11
Drugs metabolised by CYP2D6

Class of drug	Drug
Antipsychotic	Haloperidol, zuclopenthixol, thioridazine, risperidone, sertindole
Antidepressant	Amitriptyline, nortriptyline, imipramine, desipramine, clomipramine, mianserin
Analgesic	Codeine, dextromethorphan
β-blocker	Propranolol, metoprolol
Stimulant	Amphetamine (including ecstasy)

Some combinations of the above drugs are contraindicated; for other combinations reduction of the dose of antipsychotic may be required.

chotics.[157] In Caucasian populations, 7% lack functional enzyme activity and are therefore termed poor metabolizers. Several different mutations have been characterized which, in the homozygous state, cause a lack of functional enzyme activity.[158] It is possible to genotype individuals for these mutations and hence predict whether or not they will be poor metabolizers. CYP2D6 is also an important site of drug–drug interactions (Table 11).

CYP1A2

About 14% of the Caucasian population appears to be deficient in CYP1A2 activity. These individuals may be identified by a functional assay using caffeine (a substrate for CYP1A2). There also seems to be significant inter-ethnic variation, with Japanese subjects showing significantly lower enzyme capacity.[153]

CYP1A2 capacity is reduced in the elderly and increased in women as compared with men. As it is induced by *cigarette smoking* and some conventional antipsychotics are significantly metabolized by CYP1A2, cigarette smoking increases the clearance of fluphenazine and haloperidol by 100% and at least 50% respectively. Thus, smokers may require higher doses than non-smokers.

Similarly, olanzapine clearance is increased in males (by about 30%) and in smokers, and decreased in the elderly. Furthermore, if a patient ceases smoking while maintaining a constant dose of antipsychotic, they may be more at risk of adverse effects.

CYP3A4

Many conventional antipsychotics, clozapine and sertindole are also significantly metabolized by CYP3A4. This enzyme is induced by *carbamazepine*; for most conventional antipsychotics twice as much antipsychotic is required to achieve the same plasma concentration in the presence of carbamazepine as in the absence of carbamazepine. This interaction is relevant for those cases where mood stabilizers are used in conjunction with antipsychotics (for example schizoaffective psychosis).

Other substances inhibit metabolism at CYP3A4. Clozapine toxicity has been reported after the coadministration of erythromycin.[159] Individuals who are CYP2D6 poor metabolizers or who are in receipt of drugs which inhibit CYP2D6 metabolism would be expected to be at increased risk of effects secondary to interactions at CYP3A4. Sertindole is subject to clinically significant interactions at both CYP2D6 and CYP3A4.

Deep compartment washout

Chronic dosage leads to a fourth phase in drug clearance known as deep compartment washout. Urinary metabolites may be detected up to 3 months after the discontinuation of chronically dosed phenothiazines;[160] this deep compartment effect is likely to be even greater for depot preparations and may contribute to the delay in relapse seen on cessation of a depot preparation as compared to cessation of an equivalent dose of oral antipsychotic.

Variables influencing pharmacokinetic factors

The variables influencing the pharmacokinetics of antipsychotics are summarized as follows:

- age: reduction in clearance, but increased variance in clearance
- comorbid medical conditions: reduction in clearance due to reduced liver function; increased free drug concentration if plasma protein binding reduced
- genetics: polymorphic cytochrome P450 system
- drug interactions: prescribed drugs may interact at specific P450s; drugs of abuse may also affect P450 capacity

Prescribing for a first episode of schizophrenia-like psychosis

5

It is important to begin treatment as soon as possible after identifying an individual as psychotic. Reasons for prompt prescribing include the following:

- alleviation of mental suffering of the affected individual
- prevention of further deterioration in mental state with associated danger to him/herself and others (an assessment of risk must be made)
- the longer the duration of untreated psychosis, the longer is the time taken to respond to treatment and the greater the risk of future relapse[5,10,161]

This chapter considers the use of antipsychotics for first-onset cases of psychosis in which the diagnosis is a schizophrenia spectrum disorder (ie schizophrenia, schizoaffective or schizophreniform disorder). Antipsychotics are also often useful in affective psychoses (Chapter 6).

Decades of clinical experience with antipsychotics indicate that they can reduce the positive symptoms of schizophrenia. Sixty per cent of those presenting with an acute episode of schizophrenia improve to the extent that they achieve a complete remission or experience only mild symptoms when treated with antipsychotic medication for 6 weeks, compared to only 20% of patients treated with placebo.[162]

The outcome is even better for patients in their first episode. Lieberman and colleagues have demonstrated that some 83% of first-onset cases will remit by one year of treatment (Figure 2);[163] however, with each succeeding episode, the proportion who respond falls and the length of time to response also increases.

Which antipsychotic?

All the first-line antipsychotic drugs may be used in individuals suffering from their first episode of psychosis, whatever the cause. Details about the drugs are given in Chapter 4. Since there is no conclusive evidence that any particular antipsychotic is more effective than others against positive symptoms, the choice is generally made in terms of the side-effect profile of the drugs. Knowledge of the different drugs and

their adverse effects can therefore enable appropriate and safe prescribing. Patient factors influencing choice of antipsychotic include:

- age
- sex
- degree of agitation, sleep disturbance or anxiety
- concomitant depression
- relevant family history

It is important to take the age of the patient into account. For example, owing to the high risk of a dystonic reaction in young first-onset cases (especially males), antipsychotics from the group of piperazine phenothiazines (eg trifluoperazine) should be used with extreme caution in a young person presenting with a psychotic episode for the first time. Since such a dystonic event is very likely to alienate the patient and jeopardize subsequent compliance, it is better to avoid such drugs in first-onset cases. At the other end of the age range, one would tend to avoid the use of adjuvant anticholinergic drugs or even antipsychotics with pronounced antimuscarinic properties since an exacerbation of the psychosis akin to an atropine-like psychosis may occur in the elderly.

On the other hand, effects which are generally disadvantageous can sometimes

Figure 2
Cumulative percentage of first-episode patients responding to treatment. Adapted from Lieberman JA et al.[163] With permission from Elsevier Science.

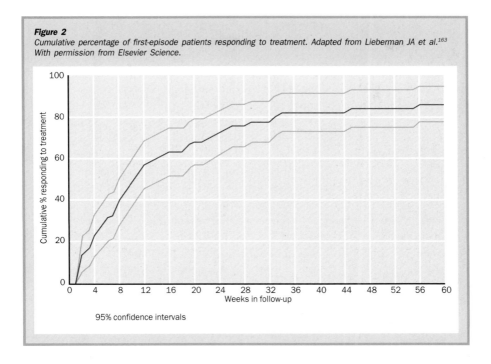

be used to advantage. Thus, sedation may be desirable in psychotic patients with prominent sleep disturbance or in acutely anxious or disturbed patients. In such cases, one might select either chlorpromazine or thioridazine from among the typicals, or olanzapine or quetiapine from among the atypical drugs. Some antipsychotics, eg risperidone, flupenthixol, olanzapine, and ziprasidone, may have a higher antidepressant activity than others, and may therefore

be appropriate in cases of psychosis accompanied by symptoms suggestive of depression.

Alternatively, an antipsychotic with low sedative effect may be combined with a sedative (eg a benzodiazepine), and the sedative withdrawn after the sleep disturbance or agitation has been resolved.

If a patient is a candidate for the depot form of maintenance medication, the oral form of the preferred depot may be the logical choice. If there is a family history of psychotic illness, and it is known which pharmacological agent was effective for the affected family member, then it is worth trying this agent as first-line medication.

Typical or atypical

Owing to the risk of agranulocytosis (0.7% in the first year[164]), clozapine has to be administered with regular haematological monitoring and cannot be prescribed as first-line treatment in most Western countries.

The other atypicals do not have this restriction and many investigators believe that, in comparison to typical antipsychotics, they are more effective and have a more favourable side-effect profile; this appears to translate to a lower drop-out rate, ie improved compliance.[112] These three properties arguably make them highly indicated for first-episode cases. In schizophrenia, the deterioration process, if it occurs, tends to be during the prepsychotic period and the first 5 years after the initial episode.[165] There may be an active pathophysiological process that underlies the active psychosis; if this can be halted during this time, then a degree of permanent deterioration may be

avoided. Evidence in support of this comes from studies indicating that effective treatment of the initial episode of illness can improve the level of recovery and long-term outcome of patients with schizophrenia.[5,161,165] Further relevant points in this argument are that atypical antipsychotics may alleviate negative symptoms to a greater extent than typical antipsychotics, and some may impair cognitive function less than typicals,[166] and may lead to a greater improvement in the quality of life.[167] They also have a lower tendency to induce EPS including TD.

Against the above it has been argued that any demonstrated superiority of atypicals over traditional drugs is simply a function of the fact that too high doses of traditional antipsychotics were used.[168] For example, in a large international double-blind study, risperidone at doses of 1 to 16 mg per day was compared with haloperidol at 10 mg per day;[169] similarly, olanzapine at doses of 2.5 to 17.5 mg/day has been compared with haloperidol at doses of 5 to 20 mg/day.[167]

Moreover, the atypicals are more expensive than the typicals, and this has limited their availability. However, there is some evidence that they may be more cost-effective.[170-172] Studies are currently in progress regarding the cost-effectiveness of using an atypical antipsychotic

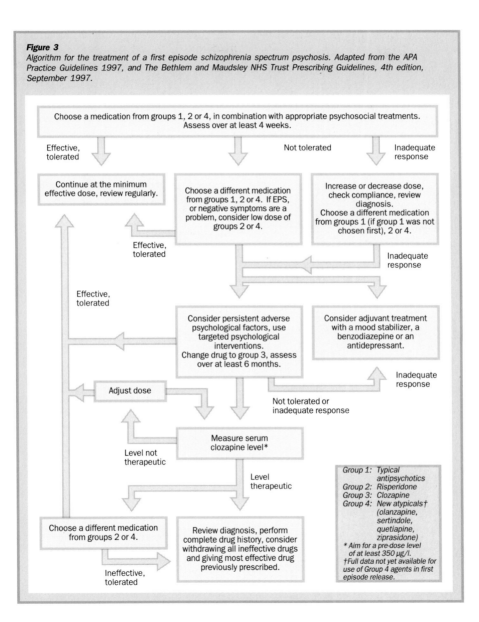

Figure 3
Algorithm for the treatment of a first episode schizophrenia spectrum psychosis. Adapted from the APA Practice Guidelines 1997, and The Bethlem and Maudsley NHS Trust Prescribing Guidelines, 4th edition, September 1997.

as first-line treatment. It may be that in the long run the short-term prescribing expense is more than offset by the gain in patient quality of life and hence reduction in morbidity-associated costs.

An algorithm for the treatment of a first episode schizophrenia spectrum psychosis is provided in Figure 3.

What dose?

D_2 receptor occupancy

It has become apparent that many first-onset patients have been prescribed too

high doses of antipsychotics. PET studies indicate that the relationship between plasma level and D_2-receptor occupancy is hyperbolic (Figure 4).[168] Doses of typical antipsychotics producing less than 60% D_2 occupancy lie on the linear portion of the curve, and tend to be associated with an inadequate clinical response. Doses corresponding to occupancies of 70–89% lie on the flatter part of the curve, with doses in the higher portion of this range tending to produce acute EPS. It has been estimated that 2 mg haloperidol produces approximately 60% D_2 occupancy.[168]

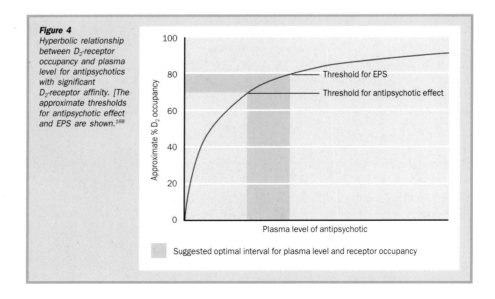

Figure 4
Hyperbolic relationship between D_2-receptor occupancy and plasma level for antipsychotics with significant D_2-receptor affinity. [The approximate thresholds for antipsychotic effect and EPS are shown.[168]

Clinical studies

Do clinical studies support the above theoretical dose ranges? It has been shown that 5 mg haloperidol daily is effective in the treatment of schizophrenia.[173] In an early fixed-dose study,[174] three doses of chlorpromazine (200 mg, 400 mg and 600 mg) were compared over 4 weeks, and it was found that in the 200 mg group there were more drop-outs due to insufficient efficacy, while EPS and other side-effects were more frequently observed in the patients taking 600 mg. The results of 19 controlled trials showed that after 2 to 10 days' treatment, there was an overall 50% response rate to less than 250 mg of chlorpromazine equivalents (see Table 12 for equivalent doses of other antipsychotics), a 56% response rate to 300–600 mg chlorpromazine equivalents and a 38% response rate to doses greater than 800 mg chlorpromazine equivalents, with more side-effects being experienced in the third group.[175] The data group therefore showed that the response rate in the medium-dose group was the best, with a lower response rate in the low- and high-dose groups, with the additional disadvantage of more adverse effects in the high-dose group.

Low doses for first-onset patients

It should be remembered, however, that these studies were carried out on mixed groups of schizophrenic patients, and that lower doses would probably be sufficient for first-episode patients. Indeed, in one particular study, the mean doses of haloperidol and risperidone used after 4 weeks of treatment were 3.9 mg and 4.1 mg respectively.[176] The dose equivalency of haloperidol and risperidone is approximately 1:1. Kopala and colleagues have conducted a study regarding the effectiveness of risperidone at two different dose levels in the treatment of first-episode schizophrenia.[116] The response rate as defined by a reduction of at least 2% in total PANSS score in the low-dose (2–4 mg) group was 91%, while in the high-dose (5–8 mg) it was 27%. It was concluded that 2–4 mg of risperidone may in fact be optimal. The mean dose used in this study (17 men, 5 women) was 4.7 mg. At the higher dose range (5–8 mg), 32% of the sample developed akathisia and 17% mild parkinsonism, both of which diminished upon reduction of the dose of risperidone.

In another study,[8] for the first phase of treatment, patients were given 2 mg risperidone daily; by 4 weeks of treatment, 66% of patients had responded to this dose. Patients who had not responded by 4 weeks were then randomized to either haloperidol or risperidone. The mean dose of haloperidol used for inpatients was found to be 4 mg, that for outpatients 3 mg, with 2 mg being the most popular dose.

In a first psychotic presentation, the degree of therapeutic response to a given dose tends to be greater than in subsequent presentations and the susceptibility to adverse effects is also higher.[177] This may explain why a dose of 2 mg of haloperidol or risperidone has been found to be clinically effective, despite the expected D_2 occupancy being only 60% (occupancy levels induced by a given dose could be higher in a first episode, as D_2-receptor upregulation will not yet have occurred). It is also important to note that the above results have been obtained in centres in which intervention occurs early and is combined with other treatment modalities in order to optimize response. The aim should be to use the lowest effective dose. Those with affective symptoms may be particularly responsive to a low-dose strategy: more rapid and complete resolution is more likely in this group.[8]

The studies reviewed by Baldessarini *et al*[175] show an improved speed of response with moderate doses when compared with a low-dose regime: the proportion of patients responding to a low dose (less than 250 mg chlorpromazine equivalents daily) after 1 day was 38%, while that responding to a moderate dose (at least 300 mg chlorpromazine equivalents) was 61%. It is possible that it is the sedative rather than the antipsychotic effect of the drug which is leading to an apparently higher response rate, which could be equally achieved by using appropriate adjuvant treatment if required (eg a benzodiazepine), without the concomitant increased risk of EPS and other unpleasant side-effects.

It has been demonstrated that good remission rates and low subsequent levels of positive symptoms are possible with low doses of antipsychotics.[8] When combined with intensive psychosocial management, there is also an associated low level of negative symptoms, which is not accounted for by a low level of depression. The reduced dose and duration of antipsychotic treatment could be a factor in the reduction of (secondary) negative symptoms.

Potential advantages of a low-dose strategy:

- reduced incidence of side-effects
- increased compliance
- reduced incidence of secondary negative symptoms

A low-dose strategy is particularly appropriate for:

- first-episode psychosis with minimal treatment delay
- cases where intensive monitoring and psychosocial management are possible
- affective psychoses

An appropriate treatment protocol for first-episode psychosis would be to initiate antipsychotic treatment at a very low dose (eg 2 mg haloperidol or 100 mg chlorpromazine equivalents), with careful monitoring and intensive psychosocial intervention, aiming for the lowest effective dose. The lowest doses likely to be effective are given in Table 12. In adolescents, the elderly, or others with a reduced metabolic capacity (eg low body weight) the appropriate dose may be even lower, for example 1 mg haloperidol or equivalent. Drug interactions, concomitant substance abuse and genetic effects (eg family history of drug sensitivity) also need to be considered, and may indicate that adjustment of the dose up or down is required.

Treatment resistance

Up to 30% of first-onset cases of schizophrenia may fail to achieve remission after 6 weeks of treatment, and a proportion of these will prove to be treatment resistant. There is evidence that long-term treatment resistance is apparent within the first 2 years and should therefore be an explicit target of early intervention.[14,24]

Treatment resistance includes both those cases for which the treatment has failed to produce adequate alleviation of the symptoms (treatment refractory) and those cases in which the subject is intolerant of the adverse effects of the treatment (treatment intolerant). It has been demonstrated that patients who were refractory to average antipsychotic doses none the less had 80–85% of their D_2 receptors occupied.[177] This argues against any benefit from further increasing the dose and, some would say, in favour of changing to a different antipsychotic, preferably one with a different receptor binding profile. Such is the logic behind the recommendation to change to an antipsychotic of a different class (for example try a butyrophenone if a phenothiazine has been employed initially) or to an atypical drug.

If the problem is treatment intolerance with the first agent, especially with EPS, then it is vital to switch to an agent with a lower incidence of EPS. If negative symptoms predominate, then risperidone, olanzapine or amisulpride may be appropriate.

For patients who fail to respond to two antipsychotics of different classes at standard therapeutic doses for at least 6 weeks ('treatment-resistant schizophrenia'), the following steps should be undertaken (see Figure 3):[178]

- **Review the diagnosis.** Is the patient really psychotic? (Or could this be a case of Munchausen's syndrome for instance?) Has an organic psychosis been excluded? Are illicit drugs interfering with therapy? (Try a urine drug screen.) Are negative symptoms dominant and, if so, is the most appropriate drug being used?

- **Check compliance.** It may be useful to perform a therapeutic blood level or, for those antipsychotics with substantial D_2 blocking activity, a prolactin level.

- **Allow sufficient time for response.** Additional time on standard doses may be sufficient in some cases, if necessary increasing the level of supervision (staffing level for inpatients).

- **Consider reducing the dose slowly for a trial period.** Moderate or high doses may cause iatrogenic negative symptoms, which may decrease the apparent clinical response. Furthermore, if a patient has a deficiency in the relevant metabolizing enzyme, they may respond better to very low doses.[179]

- **Consider increasing the dose for a trial period.** There is no evidence that 'megadose therapy' is of any value but, very occasionally, it may be advisable to increase the dose to the BNF upper limit. If the therapeutic level or prolactin level is much lower than that expected for the dose prescribed, then, if compliance has been observed and documented, the possibility of hypermetabolizer status should be considered. It would then be appropriate to increase the dose gradually, monitoring for clinical response and adverse effects, checking the appropriate level regularly until a therapeutic level is reached.

- **Change the drug** to a typical of a different class or an atypical (or a different atypical if one is already used).

- **Consider persistent adverse psychosocial factors.** High expressed emotion, whether in a home or ward environment, is likely to be deleterious to recovery. For inpatients, it may be necessary to consider the immediate ward milieu, eg whether or not the provision of a single room might be therapeutic.

Table 12
Lowest doses which may be effective in first-episode schizophrenia

	Lowest effective dose (mg/day)
Typical antipsychotics	
Chlorpromazine	100
Thioridazine	100
Trifluoperazine	5
Fluphenazine	2
Haloperidol	2
Droperidol	4 (po)
Flupenthixol	3
Zuclopenthixol	20
Atypical antipsychotics	
Amisulpiride	50*
Risperidone	2
Olanzapine	5
Quetiapine	150
Sertindole	8

Data on the lowest effective dose are from first-episode studies and, where data on specific drugs are not available, predicted lowest effective dose is given by calculation of chlorpromazine equivalents.
*50 mg if negative symptoms are predominant, 300 mg to 400 mg if positive symptoms are predominant.

- **Consider specific targeted psychological interventions.** For example, for persisting hallucinations or delusions, a cognitive approach should be tried, in addition to psychological approaches which should already be in place (Chapters 7 and 8).

- **Consider adjuvant treatment.**
  Review the history for any evidence
  of an affective component (eg cyclic
  variation in symptom level) and, as
  appropriate, add a lithium or
  another mood stabilizer or an
  antidepressant (note that carbamazepine will decrease the serum
  levels of some antipsychotics, eg
  flupenthixol, by one-third). Consider
  the short-term use of benzodiazepines for agitation (eg lorazepam
  or clonazepam).
- **Consider changing the drug to
  clozapine.** Clozapine may be tried
  after the patient has failed to
  respond adequately to or tolerate
  two drugs of two different classes
  for at least 6 weeks. Inadequate
  response includes refractory negative
  symptoms.

Targeting treatment resistance early
with atypical neuroleptics and cognitive
treatment has been predicted to reduce
long-term morbidity substantially.[19]

Consolidation

Consolidation refers to the continuation
of treatment when the acute symptoms
are resolving, in order to consolidate
the response. Many clinicians would
advise continuing antipsychotic therapy
for approximately a year (minimum of
6 months) after a first psychotic
episode. However, in McGorry's first-
episode work reported to date, less than
half of the sample were still receiving
neuroleptics at 6 months.[8] One of the
reasons for this is that only 30.5% of
the sample initially met the diagnostic
criteria for schizophrenia; for those with
a diagnosis of schizophrenia or schizophreniform disorder, the aim is 6 to 12
months of antipsychotic treatment. This
may be further extended if positive
symptoms persist, and beyond that into
a period of remission to allow for
consolidation. With affective psychoses
a similar duration of therapy was aimed
for, but 6 to 9 months was probably
more common. There are therefore no
absolute guidelines as to the length of
remission into which treatment should
continue for consolidation, but a
minimum of 6 months would seem
reasonable.

Maintenance

Maintenance refers to prophylactic
treatment to reduce the risk of future
episodes. Studies regarding the relapse
rate after a first psychotic episode may
be summarized as giving a 1-year

Table 13
Principles of maintenance treatment.

Review diagnosis
Use lowest effective dose of antipsychotic
Adjuvant psychosocial approaches for relapse prevention
Ease of access to service in crisis
Prompt adjustment in dose when required

relapse rate of 15 to 35%, and a 2-year relapse rate of 30 to 60%.[180] This relapse rate is influenced by several factors, including the use of maintenance antipsychotic medication: the 2-year relapse rate in one study was 40% on maintenance medication as compared with 60% on placebo,[6] while maintenance fluphenazine reduced the 1-year relapse rate to zero in one study.[145] The fact that 40% of patients on placebo functioned well over 2 years (including reaching a superior occupational outcome) emphasizes the importance of predicting who is likely to relapse. The principles of maintenance treatment are given in Table 13.

If the diagnosis is *schizophrenia*, the benefit of *maintenance antipsychotic* medication is clear: most patients with schizophrenia will relapse upon discontinuation of treatment, at a rate of about 10% per month; medicated patients are 2 to 10 times less likely to relapse.[181] In one review of studies in which the medication of well stabilized patients with schizophrenia was discontinued it was found that 75% of patients relapsed within 6 to 24 months.[182] At the point of taking this decision it is therefore useful to have a firm opinion regarding the diagnosis. For a predominantly affective psychosis, the appropriate maintenance medication would be a mood stabilizer.

Baldessarini *et al* reviewed the result of 33 randomized controlled trials in which high doses (mean 5200 mg/day chlorpromazine equivalents) were compared to moderate doses (mean 400 mg/day chlorpromazine equivalents).[175] The moderate doses were more effective in two-thirds of the trials, and in 95% of the studies the high doses resulted in greater neurological side-effects. Studies comparing low doses (eg 5 to 10 mg fluphenazine decanoate fortnightly) with standard doses (25 to 50 mg fluphenazine decanoate fortnightly) indicate that the low dose regime may be as effective, associated with greater improvement in instrumental and interpersonal role performances at 2 years and also with fewer EPS and signs of early TD.[162] Compliance rates with a low dose regime may also be higher.[183]

Table 14
Lowest dose of depot antipsychotics likely to be effective (with treatment interval) and range of equivalent doses.

Depot antipsychotic	Lowest effective dose	Range of equivalent doses
Flupenthixol decanoate	20 mg 2/52	20–40 mg 2/52
Fluphenazine decanoate	12.5 mg 2/52	2–25 mg 2/52
Haloperidol decanoate	50 mg 4/52	25–100 mg 4/52
Zuclopenthixol decanoate	100 mg 2/52	80–200 mg 2/52

An international consensus conference recommended that the antipsychotic dose should be reduced 20% every 6 months until a minimal maintenance dose is reached, considered to be as low as 50 mg haloperidol decanoate monthly.[184] The lowest dose of depot formulation likely to be effective is given in Table 14. The range of equivalent doses is also given; interindividual variation in metabolism means that there is a range of dose equivalencies.

In principle, the lowest effective dose to prevent relapse should be used. Undertreatment, with the high personal and possible social morbidity associated with a relapse, is as undesirable as overtreatment. It may be possible to employ a very low maintenance dose *effectively* if psychosocial approaches to relapse prevention are also employed, together with early detection of prodromal signs by patients and/or their carers, and access to a clinical service for assessment and prompt increase of the antipsychotic dose if indicated.

An intermittent maintenance approach

McGorry *et al* made the point that in a group of young people with no prior exposure to mental health services, relatively good or complete recovery, and significant levels of (partially adaptive) denial, a flight into health is common.[8] Many are determined to cease medication, yet often willing to remain in some degree of clinical contact. The team's preference, in a 'consumer-orientated approach' was to go along with their clients' desires, especially as there is a subgroup who will never relapse and who, by implication, would not need maintenance medication, but for which clear predictive indicators are not yet available.

After gradual reduction, consolidation and complete discontinuation of maintenance medication, patients are followed up closely until there are prodromal signs of a relapse, at which time the medication is reinstated. Studies regarding the efficacy of an intermittent or targeted medication approach show mixed results, which may be partly accounted for by different outcome criteria. Carpenter *et al* found an equal *rehospitalization rate* (50%) in an intermittently treated group compared with a continuously treated group during a 2-year follow-up period.[185] Herz *et al* found a nonsignificantly higher rate of re-emergence of psychotic symptoms for intermittently treated patients (30%) than for patients continuously maintained on medication (16%) over 2 years.[186] Jolley *et al* found a significant difference in the rates of psychotic symptoms between intermittently treated (30%) and continuously treated (7%) groups.[187] However, in the latter study, over 70% of the relapses were preceded by prodromal dysphoric and neurotic symptoms; the authors therefore suggested that targeted medication may be appropriate for those who relapse gradually, while retaining insight and compliance in the prodromal phase. Jolley and colleagues also found significantly fewer EPS and a trend towards less TD after 1 year in patients treated intermittently.[187]

Intermittent treatment starting *early* during a schizophrenic relapse (ie when prodromal signs are evident) is an option for patients for whom the following applies:[188]

- there was only one episode of positive symptoms
- there were no symptoms during the period of consolidation of treatment
- the patients are not keen to take continuous maintenance medication but agree to regular follow-up
- the working diagnosis is drug-induced psychosis: the psychosis may never recur if abstinence from the illicit agent is maintained

A targeted medication strategy in combination with a low-dose maintenance regime may be suited to some first-episode patients.[189] For first-onset patients who go on to experience multiple nonaffective psychotic episodes (several episodes in close proximity in the initial presentation), continuation of maintenance antipsychotic medication for at least 5 years has been advised.[162]

Practicalities of maintenance treatment

The formulation of the maintenance antipsychotic should be considered. Depot preparations have some advantages, including the potential to eliminate covert noncompliance,[190] but may be experienced as painful and demeaning and, particularly if inappropriately administered, may be associated with local complications such as nodule formation and possibly a higher incidence of TD. A low-dose oral atypical may prove to be equally effective as a maintenance agent as a depot typical, particularly those for which the half-life allows a once-daily dose regime (eg risperidone in most cases, and olanzapine or sertindole).

Combating adverse effects

Extrapyramidal side-effects (EPS)

These include parkinsonism, dystonia, dyskinesia and akathisia, with acute and tardive variants of the last three. Acute forms occur during the first days or weeks of antipsychotic administration, are dose dependent and are reversible upon antipsychotic dose reduction or discontinuation.

EPS:

- are unpleasant to experience
- may be functionally disabling
- may be distressing for family or friends to observe
- may counteract the therapeutic effect of antipsychotics
- may deter social integration
- are associated with poor compliance.

It is therefore important to avoid or limit the development of EPS as far as possible.

Acute dystonia

This describes involuntary movements with sustained muscle contraction, causing contorting, twisting, repetitive movements or abnormal postures, most commonly affecting the muscles of the head and neck.[191] Risk factors include:

- young age
- male gender
- high-potency typical antipsychotic
- high dose of typical antipsychotic
- intramuscular administration

Acute dystonia is distressing and frightening and patients will therefore tend to complain spontaneously. Nevertheless, the dystonia may be misdiagnosed or misinterpreted as dissociative phenomena, malingering or even as an attempt to persuade the doctor to prescribe anticholinergics (for their 'lift' effect). More subtle forms of dystonia, such as difficulties in speaking, chewing or swallowing, go unnoticed by staff and therefore untreated. An acute dystonia should be treated urgently, with an intramuscular anticholinergic.

Parkinsonism

Drug-induced parkinsonism resembles idiopathic Parkinson's disease, which is characterized by the triad of bradykinesia, rigidity and tremor, except that the classical pill-rolling tremor is less common in the drug-induced form. Mild rigidity may be detectable only on activation (the subject is asked to actively move the opposite limb). Bradykinesia (slow movement) may be accompanied by bradyphrenia (slow thinking), which may make it very difficult to differentiate from the negative symptoms of schizophrenia or a secondary depression. Should parkinsonism arise, where possible the drug should be changed to an

atypical; if this is not possible, dose reduction and anticholinergic medication as required should be administered.

Dyskinesia

Acute drug-induced dyskinesia refers to abnormal involuntary drug-induced movements, particularly orofacial. Of note is spontaneous or idiopathic orofacial dyskinesia, which is indistinguishable from drug-induced acute or tardive dyskinesia, seen in 5–15% of elderly individuals who have never received antipsychotic drugs.[144]

Akathisia

This is an inner sensation of dysphoria with restlessness, with an urge to move various parts of the body, manifest, for example, as rocking from to foot when standing, or an inability to sit still (if severe, patients are unable to stand without pacing).[191] Such symptoms are commonly misdiagnosed as symptoms of the psychiatric illness, which may partly account for the wide variation in reported incidence figures. It is associated with noncompliance with treatment,[192] and with aggressive and suicidal behaviour.[193] Parkinsonism is significantly

associated with akathisia; hence drugs
with a low tendency to induce
Parkinsonism also tend to have a lower
risk of akathisia. Risk factors include:

- high D_2 receptor potency
- high dose
- rapid escalation of dose

Akathisia is unfortunately less responsive to treatment than parkinsonism or
dystonia. If present, the dose of the
antipsychotic should be reduced (preferably gradually) and a switch made to
an atypical drug with a low potential to
induce the effect such as sertindole;
other agents, for example propranolol
(at 30 to 90 mg/day) may be tried if
this is not possible. Benzodiazepines
may also be helpful, especially if the
diagnosis (akathisia or psychotic agitation) is uncertain.

Sedation

Sedation is the most common single
side effect of antipsychotic medication,
especially in the initial stage of treatment. For agitated patients, the sedation
may be therapeutic; however, if
sedation persists beyond the period of
acute psychosis and causes daytime
drowsiness, it becomes a problem.

Treatment options include:

- reduce the dose
- if the drug is given in divided doses,
  give the major portion of the dose
  nocte
- use a sedative in combination with
  a non-sedative antipsychotic, so that
  the sedative can be reduced as
  necessary
- if the half-life of the drug allows,
  give it as a single nocte dose
- change to a less sedative drug

Low-potency typical antipsychotics are
more sedative than the high-potency
ones. Risperidone has a relatively low
incidence of sedation,[169] olanzapine
causes sedation in 12 to 39% of
cases.[167]

Endocrine and sexual dysfunction

Raised prolactin can be seen in association with the use of most antipsychotics as a result of blocking the
inhibitory actions of dopamine on the
anterior pituitary lactotrophs. Hyperprolactinaemia is reversible on stopping
medication.

Erectile dysfunction occurs in
23–54% of men on antipsychotics.

Other side-effects affecting sexual function include ejaculatory disturbances in men and loss of libido or anorgasmia in women and men; these are thought to be due to antiadrenergic and antiserotonergic effects, and possibly hyperprolactinaemia. In addition, specific antipsychotics (eg thioridazine and risperidone) may cause retrograde ejaculation. Twenty per cent of males on sertindole in trials had reduced or no ejaculate.[141]

Dose reduction or discontinuation (if feasible) of the medication usually results in alleviation of the symptoms. Imipramine at 25–50 mg may be helpful for treating retrograde ejaculation. If dose reduction or a switch to an alternative medication is not feasible, yohimbine (an α_2 antagonist) or cyproheptadine (a 5-HT$_2$ antagonist) may be helpful.[162]

Weight gain

Weight gain occurs with most typical antipsychotics, in up to 40% of cases, and with olanzapine and clozapine particularly commonly. Data on risperidone and sertindole indicate an average gain in weight of 1–4 kg over the first 6–8 weeks of treatment.[194] Weight gain usually plateaus during the first year of treatment and should be managed by dietary control (preferably initiated early on in treatment). There are some claims that amisulpride and ziprasidone may be less likely to produce weight gain.

Peripheral autonomic effects

The anticholinergic effects of antipsychotic medication (along with the effects of anticholinergic antiparkinsonian medication when concurrently administered) can produce a variety of adverse effects, including dry mouth, blurred vision, constipation, tachycardia, urinary retention and impaired cognitive function. These can occur in one form or another in 10–50% of treated patients, especially with agents with high muscarinic antagonism. Most reduce in severity with increased time and are treated symptomatically (eg by increased fluid intake or a high fibre diet for constipation). Anticholinergic side-effects may be particularly troublesome or dangerous in the elderly.

Many antipsychotics at high doses prolong the QT interval, which puts the individual at risk of ventricular fibrillation, especially of the Torsades de Pointes type (hence the need for cardiovascular monitoring for doses above the BNF range).

Adrenoreceptor blockade can lead to miosis, nasal stuffiness, orthostatic hypotension and priapism or inhibition of ejaculation. Orthostatic hypotension should be managed by rising slowly from a seated or lying position and possibly increasing dietary salt intake. Tachycardia may be an anticholinergic effect, or may occur secondary to orthostatic hypotension; if severe, a low-dose peripherally acting β-blocker may be used (eg atenolol). Thioridazine and clozapine have the greatest adrenoreceptor antagonist activity.

Central autonomic effects

Antipsychotics can disturb thermoregulation, leading to failure of physiological control of body temperature independent of ambient temperature. There is therefore a risk of heat stroke in hot climates and hypothermia in cold climates. Central anticholinergic toxicity can lead to impaired memory and cognition, confusion, delirium, somnolence and hallucinations. Cessation of treatment usually results in reversal of symptoms; if symptoms are severe try changing to an antipsychotic with low anticholinergic effects, eg. risperidone.

Gastrointestinal and hepatic effects

Low-potency typical antipsychotics may cause an elevation of liver enzymes and cholestatic jaundice (the latter occurs in 0.1–0.5% of patients taking chlorpromazine). Jaundice usually occurs within the first month of treatment and requires discontinuation of treatment, investigation for other causes of jaundice and substitution of another agent with a lower likelihood of inducing this complication. Olanzapine can cause a transient rise in liver enzymes but this rarely persists or necessitates stopping the drug. Risperidone may cause nausea and abdominal pain.

Miscellaneous effects

Photosensitivity can occur, particularly with low-potency typical antipsychotics; patients should be instructed to avoid excessive sunlight and/or use a UVB screen. Patchy hyperpigmentation and blue-grey discolouration may also occur. Urticaria may occur as a manifestation of phenothiazine sensitivity.

Rare but serious adverse events

Neuroleptic malignant syndrome (NMS)

Neuroleptic malignant syndrome is a rare but potentially lethal condition. It is characterized by rigidity, hyperthermia, autonomic disturbance and fluctuations in conscious level. The autonomic disturbance may include fluctuations of blood pressure, irregularities of heart rate and rhythm, loss of sphincter control, hyperpyrexia and muscle stiffness profuse sweating and sialorrhea,[195] and waxing and waning of conscious level or coma.

The changes in conscious level may lead to intermittent confusion or, in severe cases, coma. It can be sudden and unpredictable in onset, is frequently misdiagnosed and is fatal in 5–20% of cases if untreated. It usually occurs early in the course of treatment, often within the first week, or after the dose has been increased. Leucocytosis and an increase in serum creatinine kinase are usually seen. The prevalence ranges between 0.001% and 1%.[196] Risk factors include:

* young
* male
* high-potency medication
* rapid escalation of dose
* intramuscular administration

* pre-existing neurological disorder
* physical illness
* dehydration

Treatment involves discontinuation of the antipsychotic, with supportive treatment for the fever and cardiovascular symptoms (antipyretic, cardiovascular monitoring and fluid replacement as required); if severe, the patient should be transferred to an intensive care unit. Dantrolene, which reduces muscular rigidity and therefore allows core temperature to fall, may be used. The patient's mental state may be treated with benzodiazepines or ECT if required. The NMS should be clearly recorded in the patient's notes, and antipsychotics of the same class as the precipitating drug avoided. An antipsychotic of another class may be gradually introduced on recovery.

Seizures

Antipsychotic medications, particularly the low-potency typical antipsychotics and clozapine, can lower the seizure threshold. The frequency of seizures is dose related; the rates are less than 1% for all typicals at standard doses. Risk factors for medication-induced seizures include:

- idiopathic epilepsy
- head injury
- family history of epilepsy
- history of previous medication-induced seizure
- high rate of increase of dose

EEG abnormalities may be detectable before an observable seizure occurs. If a seizure occurs, the dose of drug should be reduced and a neurological examination performed. If an anticonvulsant is administered, in the case of clozapine, valproate is preferred (carbamazepine has a higher associated risk of leucopenia than valproate); it may not be advisable to prescribe clozapine at doses greater than 600 mg without anticonvulsant cover. Risperidone, olanzapine and sertindole do not show an increased seizure risk above that associated with haloperidol or placebo.

Haematological effects

The typical antipsychotics are all associated with a variety of blood dyscrasias, including a 0.08% risk of agranulocytosis.[197] The risk of agranulocytosis for patients who have been on clozapine for longer than a year is 0.07%,[164] clearly similar to the above. However, owing to the elevated risk of agranulocytosis (0.7%) in the first year of treatment and the occurrence of eight fatalities due to this in the 1970s which led to the withdrawal of clozapine from many countries until there was convincing evidence of its superior efficacy in treatment-resistant schizophrenia.[198] Mandatory haematological monitoring is associated with the prescription of clozapine.

Pigmentary retinopathies and corneal opacities

These can occur with chronic administration of the low-potency medications thioridazine and chlorpromazine, particularly at high doses (>800 mg/day). Therefore if this dose level is necessary, patients should have ophthalmological examinations every 6 months.

Chronic adverse effects

Chronic or tardive forms of EPS occur after months or years of treatment (often in the absence of a recent change in drug or dose), are not clearly dose dependent and may persist after discontinuation of medication. It may be particularly difficult to differentiate

between tardive forms of EPS and
spontaneous abnormal involuntary
movements which are intrinsic to the
schizophrenic illness. Their relevance to
the treatment of first-onset cases is not
that they are particularly likely to occur
in the short term, but rather that it is
important to prescribe in such a fashion
as to minimize the risk that they will
occur later. Furthermore, patients and
their relatives may know of the risk and
be very worried about their possible
occurrence, with predictable effects on
compliance.

Late-onset, persistent dystonia
(tardive dystonia) may be seen in
patients on chronic antipsychotic treatment with young patients being at
greatest risk for this.[199]

Tardive dyskinesia is an abnormal
involuntary movement disorder caused
by sustained exposure to antipsychotics
which can affect any part of the body,
but most commonly affects the orofacial
area. This appears as a protrusion or
twisting of the tongue, repetitive
pursing or sucking movements of the
lips, chewing and lateral movements of
the jaw or puffing of the cheeks.
Involuntary limb movements appear
choreiform or choreo-athetoid, including
athetosis of the extremities and
purposeless, stereotyped movements.
Risk factors include:[200,201]

- long duration of antipsychotic use
- high potency antipsychotic
- subtle movement disorder prior to
  treatment
- cognitive impairment
- history of alcohol abuse
- older age
- concurrent medical condition (eg
  diabetes)

Early identification of cases is the best
policy for the prevention of tardive
dyskinesia and patients on antipsychotics
for more than 4 weeks should therefore
be evaluated regularly. If dyskinesia is
present, a neurological examination to
exclude causes other than tardive dyskinesia should be conducted. Once these
have been excluded, the dose of the
antipsychotic should be gradually
reduced by 50% over 12 weeks. This
will often lead to a decrease or remission
of the tardive dyskinesia, although
withdrawal dyskinesia (initial increase in
symptoms on dose reduction or
withdrawal) may occur in some patients.
With sustained medication exposure
without dose reduction after the development of tardive dyskinesia, the likelihood
of reversibility diminishes.
Discontinuation of medication should be
considered, changing the antipsychotic to
an atypical with a very low incidence of
tardive dyskinesia, such as clozapine.[202]

There are no obvious differences in the motor phenomena of acute and tardive akathisia, although the accompanying subjective sense of restlessness may be less marked in the latter. A similar treatment approach should be employed.

Prescribing for a first episode of affective psychosis

6

The acute affective psychoses include mania, mixed mania and depression, psychotic depression and schizoaffective psychosis. Antipsychotics, benzodiazepines or antidepressants may be required. The other main drugs employed are mood stabilizers, which may be used in the acute episode and (if indicated) in prophylaxis following recovery from a first episode of mania.

Antipsychotics

Antipsychotics are commonly used in first episodes of affective psychosis. Comparisons with lithium suggest that antipsychotics are less effective in stabilizing mood, but have a more rapid effect on manic excitement.[203]

The principles of the use of antipsychotics are outlined in Chapters 4 and 5. However, since their sedative properties are at least as valuable in the treatment of acute mania as their antipsychotic properties, it may well be preferable to use a drug

with well-established sedative properties, such as chlorpromazine.
Furthermore, it may be necessary to
use larger doses in the short term to
control severe elation or disturbed
behaviour than would be used in the
care of a patient with a first episode of
a clearcut schizophrenic nature. Since
such doses carry with them a significant risk of side-effects (Chapter 4), it
may be advisable to attempt to
minimize the dose required by the
adjunctive use of a benzodiazepine or
mood stabilizer.

It should also be remembered that
antipsychotics may provoke depression,[204] and therefore one should be
alert for patients switching from mania
to profound depression.[205] Here again
the addition of a mood stabilizer may
be valuable.

Benzodiazepines

Benzodiazepines are useful in the treatment a first psychotic episode, not on
their own but together with an antipsychotic or mood stabilizer. Adjunctive
use of benzodiazepines is appropriate
for patients with:

- severe agitation
- severe comorbid anxiety

If a benzodiazepine is used together
with an antipsychotic, the dose of
antipsychotic required may be less (at
higher doses of antipsychotic, the gain
in clinical effect is mainly in terms of
sedation, with little gain in antipsychotic effect, see Chapter 5, which can
equally be provided by a benzodiazepine).

The use of lorazepam and
clonazepam in acute mania is supported
by some small double-blind studies.[205]
Indeed, Chouinard reported that
clonazepam had some advantages over
lithium in such adjunctive treatment of
acute mania in a double-blind,
crossover study.[206] Lorazepam has a
shorter half-life and may be more effective than clonazepam in very acute
disturbance or severe agitation;[207,208] it
can be given as 1–4 mg orally or IM,
repeated every 2–6 hours as required to
a maximum of 4 mg daily. Clonazepam
may be given as 0.5–2 mg orally every
2–6 hours up to 6 mg. After brief
courses (2–6 weeks) of benzodiazepines,
most patients tolerate gradual dose
reduction without exhibiting signs of
dependency.

Contraindications to the use of
benzodiazepines in first-episode
psychosis include:

- previous benzodiazepine-induced

dysphoria or behavioural disturbance
• sedative abuse

Antidepressants

Antidepressants should be prescribed as
appropriate for a first episode of
psychosis in which depressed mood
predominates. However, one must be
cautious since in a proportion of cases
such a depressive episode will be the
first presentation of a bipolar affective
disorder, and the use of all types of
antidepressants has been associated with
the precipitation of hypomania or
mania in bipolar illness. The likelihood
of this occurring is reported to be lower
for selective serotonin reuptake
inhibitors (SSRIs) than for tricyclic
antidepressants.[209]

In a patient where a switch into
mania appears a significant risk (for
example where there is a strong family
history of mania), this risk may be
minimized by the prescription of a
mood stabilizer.

Mood stabilizers

The main mood stabilizers which may
be considered for use in a first episode
of affective psychosis are lithium, carbamazepine and valproate.

Lithium

The overall response rate to lithium in
four placebo-controlled studies of lithium
in acute mania on a total of 116 patients
was 78%.[210] Despite this, lithium is now
rarely used alone in the treatment of
acute mania because there is a delay of
several days in the onset of its effect,
and it takes 2 to 3 weeks to approach
full effect. Therefore, most clinicians,
faced with a first episode of mania,
would initially use antipsychotic drugs.

Many clinicians combine lithium with
an antipsychotic. There were early
reports suggesting a toxic interaction
between lithium and typical antipsychotics (particularly haloperidol in high
doses[211,212]) causing a clinical syndrome
resembling both lithium toxicity and
neuroleptic malignant syndrome. A
subsequent series demonstrated the
safety of combining haloperidol (up to
30 mg daily) with lithium at levels of
up to 1 mEq/l.[213] Therefore, the combination can be used provided blood
levels are maintained below this level;
should any neurological symptoms be
noted, lithium should be temporarily
discontinued.[214]

Lithium may be used by itself where there is reason to avoid antipsychotics (for example where the patient or family objects or there are severe side-effects). Lithium works best in patients with pure, relatively mild mania.[215] Many first-episode cases of mania fall into this category, and it is in those patients in whom the use of lithium alone may be most valuable.

Patients with more severe mania (marked overactivity and delusions), significant depression or dysphoria, EEG abnormalities or a negative family history of mood disorder are less likely to respond to lithium alone. In such cases, antipsychotics should be prescribed either as monotherapy or with a mood stabilizer.

Mode of action

Lithium has numerous effects on biological systems, and it is unclear which of these determine its therapeutic effects.[214] It can substitute for sodium, potassium, calcium and magnesium, entering cells via sodium and other channels, but is extruded less efficiently than sodium. The cell:plasm ratio for lithium is therefore much higher than that of sodium, and within the cell it may act on second and third messenger systems, implicated second messenger systems including G-proteins, cAMP and the phosphatidyl inositol system, and third messenger systems including kinases. It can also block the development of the dopamine receptor supersensitivity that normally occurs during prolonged treatment with dopamine-blocking (antipsychotic) drugs.[216]

Valproate

Valproate is also effective in the treatment of acute mania.[217,218] Patients with mixed affective states have been shown to benefit more from valproate than from lithium.[219,220] Valproate was also better tolerated than lithium, 11% discontinuing due to side-effects of lithium and only 6% due to side-effects of valproate.

Response usually occurs within 7–14 days of reaching a serum level of 50 mg/l, especially in mild or moderate mania; the use of a loading dose of 20 mg/kg per day may lead to an improvement in manic symptoms within 3 days.[221] Valproate is particularly useful in cases of comorbid alcohol and substance abuse (where the problems of lithium toxicity are especially likely), and in those who have not responded to lithium.

Mode of action

Valproate is thought to increase the function of the inhibitory neurotransmitter γ-aminobutyric acid (GABA); it may also enhance central serotonergic activity.[222]

Carbamazepine

Nineteen double-blind studies using various types of design (mostly crossover with either lithium or antipsychotics) demonstrated comparable efficacy of carbamazepine in mania to lithium or antipsychotics.[223] However, these studies have been criticized for their crossover design, and for the fact that they may have included an excess of lithium nonresponders. There is some delay in carbamazepine's action, but less so than with lithium, and it may be more effective than lithium in severe psychotic mania,[224] or in mixed affective states.

Mode of action

Carbamazepine reduces calcium channel (L-type) activation by depolarization and blocks the effect of glutamate at N-methyl-d-aspartate (NMDA) receptors.[214] An anti-kindling effect may underlie some of its therapeutic effects. Both lithium and carbamazepine inhibit cGMP accumulation in lymphocytes, possibly by mechanisms involving the nitric oxide second messenger system, which is stimulated by NMDA receptors.[225] Although patients who respond to valproate do not necessarily respond to carbamazepine and vice versa, there is evidence of some cross tolerance between carbamazepine and valproate,[226] indicating that there may be a degree of shared mechanism of action.

Indications for valproate or carbamazepine in first-onset affective psychosis

- Failure to respond to antipsychotics and/or lithium
- intolerance to antipsychotics and/or lithium
- severe psychotic mania
- mixed affective state or significant dysphoria
- negative family history of mood disorder
- EEG abnormalities
- comorbid substance abuse (valproate)
- abnormal renal function

Like lithium, valproate may be used together with the atypical antipsychotics. Carbamazepine is contraindicated with clozapine as it has an associated risk of blood dyscrasias and could increase the risk of clozapine-associated agranulocytosis.

Mood stabilizers as prophylactic agents following recovery from first-episode psychosis

The vast majority of patients suffering their first episode of psychosis respond readily to treatment. The question then is whether or not to suggest the use of prophylactic medication.

In the long term, prophylactic strategies which aim to reduce the severity and frequency of episodes are probably the most important aspect of the treatment of bipolar affective disorder. However, one does not wish to condemn first-episode patients to long-term prophylactic medication without being sure that the benefits outweigh the disadvantages.

After three episodes of bipolar illness a new episode can be expected within an average of a year.[227,228] The current generally accepted criterion for lithium prophylaxis is two episodes in 5 years.

However, some clinicians use lower threshold criteria: two episodes within any time frame if the second episode is severe (for example associated with a serious suicide attempt), or a single episode of mania associated with a positive family history of bipolar I.

In the authors' views, therefore, prophylactic treatment may be indicated after a first psychotic (manic) episode in a patient with a family history of severe bipolar disorder.

Similarly, it may occasionally be useful to use a mood stabilizing drug as prophylaxis after a first episode of mania which is unduly severe and prolonged, or which proceeds into severe depression. However, since such cases are the exception, only an abbreviated account of the use of mood stabilizers in prophylaxis will be given; the data, of course, refer to all cases of bipolar illness rather than first episodes.

Lithium

In a review of the ten major double-blind studies comparing lithium prophylaxis to placebo in bipolar illness, the relapse rate on lithium was seen to be 34%, compared to 81% on placebo.[210] However, there are questions over whether the benefit of lithium in ordinary clinical practice (as opposed to the artificial setting of a clinical trial) is as great.

Guscott and Taylor made the point that efficacy (the potential of a treatment, or whether it *can* work) must be distinguished from effectiveness (the results obtained under clinical conditions, or whether it *does* work).[229] The evidence regarding the efficacy of lithium has been reviewed in detail.[230,231]

It is important that patients are followed up by healthcare professionals with a high level of commitment. One possibility is in the context of an early psychosis unit, where available. An alternative setting which, in fact, most closely approximates the conditions of the early efficacy studies is the specialized lithium or mood disorders clinic.

Withdrawal of lithium

This is associated with a relapse rate in excess of the relapse rate that patients had prior to lithium treatment, especially in the first 3 months after discontinuation.[232] One study showed similar median times to 50% risk of recurrence of mania/hypomania or depression, with the polarity of the first recurrence being highly concordant (83.6%) with that of the first lifetime episode.[233] A doubling of the suicide attempt rate is seen to occur in the first year following lithium discontinuation, with the rate returning to baseline level after 1 year.[234]

Goodwin has calculated that if the risk of withdrawal mania on cessation of lithium is 50%, then it is necessary to be on lithium for at least 30 months before the net advantage is greater than the net disadvantage.[232] This implies that patients should not be prescribed lithium unless there is a high likelihood of them remaining on lithium for at least 30 months.

The excess relapse rate may be reduced by gradual as opposed to rapid discontinuation,[233,235] where gradual means discontinuing the lithium over 15 to 30 days.

Response to lithium

A number of studies have shown relapse rates in excess of 20% despite adequate blood levels.[236–239] The factors predicting good and poor response to lithium are given in Table 15.[214]

For cases in which response has been suboptimal, or there has been loss of efficacy, clinicians may be wary of discontinuing lithium for the reasons given above. Hence combination

Table 15
Factors affecting response to lithium.

Good response	Poor response
Family history of bipolar disorder	Neurological signs
Family history of response to lithium	Mixed or dysphoric mania
First episode manic	Schizoaffective
	Poor compliance
	Substance abuse
	Rapid cycling pattern

Table 15
Factors affecting response to lithium.

therapy (the addition of valproate) may be tried, or lithium may be discontinued gradually and carbamazepine introduced (possibly with an overlap period of low doses of both agents). With combination treatment the risk of side-effects of both agents is increased, hence the additional agent should be commenced gradually, titrating to response and side-effects.

Valproate

Valproate may reduce the frequency and severity of affective episodes over extended periods, including in those patients with mixed mania, bipolar II disorder, and schizoaffective disorder.[240]

It seems that valproate may be more effective in the prevention of manic and mixed episode relapses than depressive episodes, and that the drug's mood-stabilizing effects may be augmented by lithium, carbamazepine, thyroid hormone and clozapine.

The efficacy of valproate in prophylaxis is equal to or superior to lithium, with a lower incidence of intolerance to valproate. The incidence of intolerance to valproate is 10–13%, and that to lithium 22–25%.[241,242]

Carbamazepine

Fourteen controlled or partially controlled studies indicate that, overall,

63% of patients show moderate to marked response, which is a comparable response rate to that of lithium.[223] It is possible that some subgroups of patients respond better to carbamazepine than to lithium, for example those with schizoaffective disorder[224] or rapid cycling bipolar affective disorder. Like lithium and valproate, it appears to have a greater antimanic than antidepressant effect, and may lose efficacy with time, although the latter is difficult to differentiate from a spontaneous deterioration in the disorder. Studies with a mirror image design indicate that, like lithium, carbamazepine discontinuation may be associated with a withdrawal mania.

Practicalities of prescribing mood stabilizers

Patients should be given adequate information to enable them to give *informed* consent. Material produced by self help groups such as the UK Manic Depression Fellowship may be useful. It is essential to give adequate information regarding the possible adverse effects of the medication.

Table 16 shows the contraindications, appropriate investigations, therapeutic serum ranges, formulations and starting regimes for lithium, valproate and carbamazepine. Modified release (m/r) preparations will tend to give more stable blood levels over a 24-hour period than standard formulations, and are preferable for all of these agents.

Lithium

Patients should be advised regarding the need to avoid dehydration and sodium depletion. Serum lithium levels should be performed 12 hours after the last dose. The therapeutic range most often quoted is 0.6–1.0 mM.[205] A lower lithium level will tend to be associated with fewer adverse effects (including cognitive slowing), but the trade-off is a higher risk of relapse.[243]

In pregnancy, there is maximum teratogenic risk during the first trimester. If the pregnancy is planned, gradual withdrawal of lithium over the month preceding conception gives minimal risk to the foetus. Pregnancy is a time of reduced risk of psychotic relapse, whereas the postnatal period is a time of very high (up to 50%) relapse rate; lithium should be reinstated within 48 hours after childbirth. It should also be noted that lithium is contraindicated in breast-feeding. A number of important drug interactions occur (Table 17).

Table 16
Contraindications, investigations, therapeutic range, appropriate formulation and starting regime for mood stabilizers.[205,244,245]

	Lithium	Valproate	Carbamazepine
Contraindications	Impaired renal function, other causes of significant fluid or sodium imbalance, cardiac failure, recent myocardial infarction	Hepatic dysfunction (or family history of severe hepatic dysfunction), history of blood dyscrasia	Renal or hepatic impairment, cardiac arrhythmias, history of impairment, arrhythmias, history of blood dyscrasia
Investigations – pretreatment	Renal function, FBC, TFTs +/- creatinine clearance MSU, ESR BP, ECG, weight	Liver function, FBC +/- prothrombin time, renal function	FBC, liver and renal function +/- MSU, TSH, ECG, reticulocyte count
Investigations – during treatment	3-monthly BP, renal function, FBC, 6-monthly TSH, lithium level after 4–7 days, then weekly until dose constant for 4 weeks, then 3-monthly	monthly FBC, liver function 1st 6/12, then every 6 to 12/12, valproate level may be taken at frequency indicated by rapidity of dose escalation until dose adjusted	monthly FBC, liver and renal function 1st 6/12, then 6 to 12/12 with TSH, carbamazepine levels may be taken every 2–4 weeks until stable for 2–3/12
Therapeutic range of serum level	0.4–1.0 mM	50–120 mg/l	>7 mg/l
Formulation	m/r formulations preferred after acute phase	m/r formulation (sodium valproate and valproic acid)	m/r formulation
Starting regime	Varies according to preparation, see BNF	200 mg od or bd, increasing by 200 mg per 3 days up to 2000 mg according to serum level and clinical response	200 mg daily, increasing at weekly intervals up to 400 mg bd

Table 17
Significant drug interactions.

Drugs	Nature of the interaction
Diuretics (loop diuretics and thiazides), NSAIDs and ACE inhibitors	Increase lithium levels
Antacids, acetazolamide and theophylline	Reduce lithium levels
SSRIs, carbamazepine, phenytoin, sumatriptan, methyldopa, diltiazem, verapamil, erythromycin, metronidazole, metoclopramide, domperidone and antipsychotics at high lithium levels	Increase risk of neurotoxicity

Valproate

The incidence of gastrointestinal adverse effects is reduced by the use of the modified release preparation which is valproate and valproic acid combined (divalproex in the USA, *epilim chrono* in the UK). Monitoring of full blood count (especially platelets) and liver function may take place regularly until the patient is clinically stable and the valproate level is in the therapeutic range. However, the management should not rely on these investigations since clinical signs and symptoms (malaise, nausea, vomiting, easy bruising and oedema) are more reliable indicators of hepatotoxicity.[205]

Serum valproate levels should be taken immediately before the largest dose in the day (trough level). The recommended therapeutic range for serum levels (50–120 mg/l) is based on levels largely taken from studies in epilepsy. Studies in mania indicate that few patients benefit from treatment unless a level above 50 mg/l is reached.[218,246] This will usually correspond to a daily dose of at least 800 to 1000 mg.

Aspirin and fatty foods may transiently increase the percentage of the active free moiety, potentially worsening dose-related side effects.[242] Carbamazepine reduces valproate levels, while valproate increases the formation of an active metabolite of carbamazepine (see below). Cimetidine inhibits the metabolism of valproate and therefore increases the serum valproate level.

A foetal valproate syndrome has been described.

Carbamazepine

Although for epilepsy a therapeutic range of 6 to 12 mg/l is reported, a consensus opinion regarding the therapeutic range in bipolar affective disorder has not yet emerged. A review of the use of carbamazepine in bipolar affective disorder by Taylor and Duncan concluded that levels above 7 to 8 mg/l tended to be associated with efficacy, with mean daily doses ranging from 614 to 1400 mg.[244]

Carbamazepine is a teratogen (increased risk of neural tube defects); patients should be informed regarding this and regarding the potential ineffectiveness of oral contraceptives (clearance of these is increased by carbamazepine). In the event of pregnancy occurring on carbamazepine, high-dose folate (5 mg daily) should be administered and vitamin K given to mother and baby at birth.

Drug–drug interactions are a common problem with carbamazepine. Over a period of 1 to 3 months, carbamazepine induces P450 enzymes, especially CYP3A4. This means that many compounds metabolized at least partially by this pathway (including

Table 18
Drugs metabolized at least partially by CYP3A.[113,156]

Typical antipsychotics, especially haloperidol
Clozapine, sertindole
Tricyclic antidepressants
SSRIs (fluoxetine*, fluvoxamine*)
Valproate
Steroids* (oral contraceptives, prednisolone, tamoxifen, etc)
Warfarin
Antibiotics (trimethoprim, doxycycline, erythromycin*, isoniazid*)
Analgesics (dextromethorphan, dextropropoxyphene*)
Anaesthetics (lidocaine*, midazolam)
Cardiac drugs (nifedipine*, diltiazem, verapamil*, digitoxin)
Immunosuppressants (cyclosporin*, ondansetron)
Theophylline

The drugs marked with an asterisk, as well as cimetidine, inhibit the metabolism of carbamazepine.

carbamazepine itself) will have a shorter half-life. Other drugs (some of them metabolized by CYP3A4) inhibit the metabolism of carbamazepine and the other 3A4-metabolized drugs (Table 16). Valproate leads to an increase in the formation of an active (epoxide) metabolite of carbamazepine. As valproate inhibits the P450 system and carbamazepine induces this system, complex metabolic interactions may result with this combination.

Common adverse effects of mood stabilizers

Lithium

The majority of patients on lithium experience at least one side-effect.[246]

Thyroid

Increased TSH occurs in 23% of patients, goitre in 5% and clinical hypothyroidism in 5–10% (depending on dose and duration of treatment). Patients with a family history of thyroid disease or pre-existing thyroid antibodies are at greater risk. The clinical signs of hypothyroidism may easily be mistaken for depression. Lithium-induced hypothyroidism may be treated by the administration of thyroxine.

Renal effects

Polyuria and a compensatory increased thirst are noted by about one-third of patients on lithium (lithium reduces the responsiveness of the distal tubule to antidiuretic hormone, and may occasionally cause a full-blown nephrogenic diabetes insipidus.[247] This is a dose-related side-effect and, if troublesome, may therefore be managed by reducing the dose, if possible. For patients in whom a reduction in dose is not appropriate, amiloride may be used with caution. No deterioration in glomerular filtration rate occurs in the majority of patients whose lithium levels are monitored regularly; occasional cases of chronic renal failure have been attributed to lithium, which may be a rare idiosyncratic reaction to lithium. Histological change in the kidney may be found in up to 20% of patients.

Nervous system

In many patients lithium produces a fine tremor of the hands. The combination of lithium with drugs which tend to increase its CNS toxicity carries a higher risk of tremor. The tremor may change during the day and may tend to be aggravated by tiredness, anxiety, smoking or caffeine intake. It is a dose-related side-effect which tends to be reduced with the modified release formulation. If troublesome, it may be treated with a low-dose β-blocker such as propranolol (10 to 20 mg half an hour before the effect is required), but note this effect declines with repeated usage. Cerebellar tremor and inco-ordination are signs of toxicity, as are the more severe forms of fine tremor or parkinsonism. Lithium impairs neuro-muscular transmission (it exacerbates myasthenia gravis and potentiates succinylcholine); some patients may notice reduced reaction speed and preci-sion. In the first few weeks of treatment a sensation of undue fatigue may be experienced.

Cognitive effects

Patients on lithium frequently complain of an adverse effect on memory. Lithium discontinuation studies give some evidence of an objective effect on memory; some of the patients who do not relapse show improved memory for visual impressions and an increased ability to perform complicated tasks based on visual impressions and reaction ability. However, although hypomanic periods may be missed, productivity and creativity is thought by at least half of those taking lithium (including profes-sional artists) to be improved.[248]

Skin

Lithium may exacerbate acne or psoria-sis. Tetracyclines should be used with caution because of their possible inter-action with lithium, but retinoids can be used. Hair loss and altered texture may also occur in about 12% of patients, and there may be golden discolouration of the nail plates.

Metabolic effects and weight gain

About 25% of patients on long-term lithium gain more than 10 pounds in weight. This may be due to an increased consumption of calorific drinks, but also to increased food intake. Lithium also produces subtle alterations in glucose and insulin metab-olism, and may impair glucose toler-ance. Lithium can also antagonize aldosterone and increase angiotensin levels, with fluid retention and oedema. The oedema may be localized and is usually transient; it is worse with higher doses. If patients aim to lose weight through dieting, fasting, dehydration and salt deficiency should be avoided. Prevention of weight gain by advice prior to commencement of treatment is more effective than measures aimed at reducing weight.

Gastrointestinal effects

During the first 1–2 weeks of lithium treatment, nausea, abdominal cramps and loose stools (possibly with urgency of defaecation) may be experienced. Usually these symptoms soon remit; the use of divided doses or modified release preparations may assist symptom remission (occasionally modified release formulations may also cause gastrointestinal irritation).

The side-effects most commonly given as reasons for nonadherence to treatment are: polyuria and thirst, tremor, memory impairment and weight gain. In order to increase adherence, the prescriber should ask the patient about side-effects, take any reported side-effects seriously and aim for the lowest clinically effective lithium level.

Lithium intoxication, with a serum level about 1.5 mM, is a medical emergency. Its characteristics and treatment are described in detail by Schou[246] and Cookson.[214] Most cases occur as a complication of long-term therapy and are caused by reduced excretion of the drug due to:

- dehydration
- infection
- co-administration of drugs that interact

- salt deficiency
- prolonged unconsciousness
- narcosis and surgery
- pregnancy and labour

Toxicity may also be caused by an overdose of lithium, with delayed onset of symptoms (12 hours or more) due to slow entry of lithium into the tissues and continuing absorption from modified-release formulations.

Valproate

The common side-effects of valproate are all reversible and dose-dependent:

- nausea, dyspepsia, loose stools
- increased appetite, weight gain
- reversible hair loss
- thrombocytopenia, platelet dysfunction
- raised liver enzymes
- lethargy

Use of the modified-release formulation and a slow dose escalation protocol reduces the incidence of these. Gastrointestinal symptoms, weight gain and hair loss are none the less common causes of treatment discontinuation.[205] If dyspepsia is troublesome, ranitidine may help. Serum amylase should be measured in any patient who presents with acute abdominal pain. Hair loss is usually transient; some reports suggest that vitamins with trace minerals reduce this problem.[205] Regrowth may be curly. Although raised liver enzymes are not uncommon, because of the occurrence of hepatic failure, patients with raised liver function tests (LFTs) should be assessed clinically, and monitored until the LFTs return to normal. If the raised LFTs are associated with a prolongation of the prothrombin time and other signs of impending hepatic failure, valproate should be discontinued.[249]

Carbamazepine

The common side-effects of carbamazepine are:

- nausea, +/– appetite loss and abdominal pain
- ataxia, clumsiness
- dizziness or lightheadedness
- transient diplopia

Of these, nausea, blurred vision or diplopia, dizziness and unsteadiness of gait are worse during the initiation stages, dose-related and may be dose-limiting. They are reversible upon dose reduction or cessation of treatment. Nausea may be particularly troublesome, and may be minimized by taking the drug with food, using a modified-release formulation and, especially if initiated in between episodes, using a slow escalation protocol (eg 100–200 mg daily, increasing by 100–200 mg every 1–2 weeks). If the maculopapular erythematous rash occurs, this requires great caution and usually cessation of the drug. Blood dyscrasias include leucopenia, agranulocytosis, aplastic anaemia and thrombocytopenia. A moderate leucopenia occurs in up to 2% of patients and does not require cessation of therapy; life-threatening agranulocytosis and aplastic anaemia may develop suddenly in about 8 per million patients treated,[214] and require immediate cessation of the drug and urgent medical attention.

Psychosocial approaches – 1
The acute episode and its aftermath

7

The establishment and maintenance of a therapeutic alliance is of course the foundation on which any successful psychosocial intervention is based. The clinician needs to demonstrate to the patient and relatives that he or she recognizes the pattern of symptoms as evidence of a serious disturbance at the biological level and can give appropriate pharmacological treatment,[250] while also giving time to exploration of the illness model of the patient and their family. He or she also needs to act in such a consistent and caring manner as to win the trust of the patient and family.

Once a therapeutic alliance has been established, a variety of psychosocial approaches may be used, with the following overall objectives:

- to provide suitable psychoeducation for the patient, family and any significant others
- to facilitate adaptation to the psychosocial effects of the psychotic episode and modify social risk factors

- to alleviate symptoms, as an adjunct to medication
- to enhance compliance with drug treatment and generally prevent recurrence
- to promote early recognition of recurrence and appropriate intervention
- to reduce the risk of suicide

The first three of these will be discussed here in relation to the treatment of the patient during the acute psychosis and its aftermath, the last three in the next chapter. Obviously, the clinician needs to assess each individual patient and tailor the nature and extent of intervention to that patient's needs and the particular stage of the psychotic episode and the subsequent recovery. Different approaches (for example family psychoeducation or social skills training) may be complementary, leading to a better outcome than if a single approach is used alone.[251]

Provision of suitable psychoeducation

The provision of basic information regarding the illness and its treatment is a right of all psychotic patients. The cumbersome term 'psychoeducation'

refers to the technique of providing the patient and his or her family with the appropriate information about the nature and probable course of psychotic illness, the treatment options available and the resources of the healthcare and community services. The goal of psychoeducation for both patient and family is twofold: firstly, to improve their understanding of the illness itself; secondly, to modify their behaviour and attitudes.[20]

Even when acutely psychotic, patients may understand information of a *pragmatic* nature, and may find it less threatening to be given such information than to be excluded from the information flow. Of course, the information needs to be provided in a flexible way, taking into account the individual patient's background as well as experience of psychosis, so that it is comprehensible, and encourages him/her to develop an adaptive explanatory model about his/her psychotic episode.

It will often be more useful to spend time discussing individual symptoms such as delusions (often better termed as 'unusual beliefs'), hallucinations and the experience of mood swings, rather than focus on diagnosis. For instance, it may be valuable to explain that normal people can experience hallucinations (for example following the death of a loved one or in extreme stress) and that the first experience of an auditory hallucination or 'voice' is often in the context of disturbed mood.[252]

Indeed, owing to the difficulty of providing an accurate diagnosis in a first psychotic episode, it is usually better to use the general term 'acute psychotic episode', analogous to other syndromal diagnoses in medicine (eg 'cardiac failure'). More specific diagnoses (for example schizophrenic versus affective groups) may be discussed if the patient or his/her relatives inquire, but should not be emphasized unduly. If terms such as schizophrenia are used (for instance if there is a strong family history), the clinician must be careful to avoid giving an unduly pessimistic prognosis as patients and their relatives may associate this term with inevitable mental deterioration and violence. In such a situation, it may be useful to mention that approximately 75% of patients recover after a first episode of schizophrenia.[163]

It is vital to explore and understand the model of the illness that the patient and his/her family or friends hold. Once this is established, the clinician can assist patients and their families towards accepting a realistic model of the disorder with reasons for the different modes of treatment. A biopsychoso-cial vulnerability model may be used to integrate the role of adverse psychosocial factors and biological vulnerability in the generation of an acute psychotic episode.

Later, one can use this model to address the prevention of relapse by examining the role of the various precipitating elements, and devising strategies which reduce the likelihood of their recurrence. Information should be communicated in a supportive manner, with a hopeful attitude, enlisting the patient and his/her family as *collaborators* in the recovery process.

Patients, their families and any significant others are generally very distressed by the first florid manifestation of psychosis and fearful of what it portends. In the face of such a threatening event, individuals need:

• to find meaning,
• to regain mastery over their lives,
• to protect or regain self-esteem.[253]

The provision of suitable information can assist both the patient and their family in finding meaning in the episode and in regaining self-esteem.

It is also important to provide both patients and their families with adequate information concerning the likely side-effects of drugs.

It must be remembered that the needs of the patient and his/her relatives may not coincide and will vary with the stage of the illness. Indeed, it may be possible to recognize key psychological conflicts and unresolved issues within the *content* of the psychotic phenomena.[254] Although it is rarely (if ever) appropriate to utilize any such understanding in an interpretive manner at this phase of illness, displaying an active interest in these matters is therapeutic for the patient; indeed, such empathy should be part of good clinical practice.

More comprehensive psychoeducation for the patient should be deferred until the acute psychosis has responded to treatment. The rate of assimilation and acceptance of a realistic model of illness which differs from the individual's own model is influenced by several factors, including denial, symptom persistence and IQ. Denial persisting at the stage when delusions and other psychotic symptoms have abated may be protective and may therefore need to be respected: it may represent a 'healthy' resistance to the psychological threat of stigmatization.[254]

One of the main aims of psychoeducation must be to remove the feelings of shame and stigmatization which are associated with psychosis. Stigmatization may be internal, secondary to the

person's own pre-existing attitudes to the mentally ill, or it may be external, secondary to the views held by family, friends, employers and the wider society. Stigmatization may be a particular problem for patients with a high premorbid level of functioning and/or a particularly responsible job. Destigmatization may be assisted by:

- the use of normalizing information (for example that hallucinations can occur in anyone in certain circumstances)
- encouragement of a 'blame-free' acceptance of the illness
- a group format, via the process of 'universality' (ie group members having a common experience[255]
- suitable written material from patient support groups or biographical accounts

The use of a group format for psychoeducation may be particularly successful in young patients, who value autonomy and youth culture.[20]

Where denial leads to noncompliance with treatment, techniques such as compliance therapy may assist.

Those close to the patient need the chance to talk about the episode in some detail, with the opportunity to ask their questions. Emotions may run high, with unhelpful feelings of blame or self-blame. Finding the right time for this may not be easy, and it may be best done in the context of a family conference.

The clinician must always remember that his/her initial contact with the patient and family may set the tone of their attitudes to all future contact with the psychiatric services. Compulsory treatment should therefore be avoided whenever possible. Furthermore, when a patient has been subject to compulsory treatment with the agreement of the family, he or she is often filled with a sense of betrayal. In family meetings, these feelings may be explored slowly.[256]

Patients and their relatives may be afraid that a recurrence will occur with little or no warning, and they may also differ in their opinions of what would constitute a recurrence and what would be part of the patient's usual personality or within the spectrum of normal reactions to events. Such discrepancies in perceptions can lead to significant family conflict.[256]

Different levels of information may be appropriate for different families and at different stages of the illness. Significant differences have been found between families containing a member affected by bipolar affective disorder and families with a member affected by schizophrenia: the former tend to be of a higher socioeconomic status, to be more psychologically minded and more resistant to a didactic approach to treatment.[257] The media used for psychoeducation should be tailored to the individual; ideally a variety of reading material as well as videotapes and computer-assisted material should be available.[20]

Facilitation of adaption to the psychosocial effects of the psychotic episode

The treatment milieu

Wherever possible, patients suffering their first psychotic episode should be treated at home. Home-based care is less traumatic to the patient and certainly less stigmatizing, and relatives often prefer it in spite of the extra pressure it places on the rest of the family. However, hospital admission is often unavoidable especially in patients showing manic symptoms, bizarre behaviour or violence.[36]

Appropriate inpatient units

All too often in the UK and USA, teenage patients suffering their first psychotic episode are admitted to overcrowded wards with highly disturbed older patients where the threat of violence or the availability of illicit drugs make the patient worse.[30] There is no doubt that calm but sociable wards facilitate recovery,[258] and the distraught or disorganized patient may benefit from a ward environment aimed at reducing environmental chaos.[259]

Ideally, those patients requiring admission should be cared for in a unit specializing in first-onset cases. In the absence of such a unit, a meaningful activity programme in as relaxed an atmosphere as possible may be provided for inpatients away from the ward, or for outpatients, and may reduce negative symptoms, encourage the development of social skills and improve self-esteem. In such an environment, one can begin the process by which the patient gradually develops insight, acquires more appropriate coping strategies and then resumes responsibility for him/herself before being reintegrated back into the community.

Children

One should not forget that a proportion of those undergoing their first psychotic episode will be parents. Indeed, for women, the period following childbirth is the period of maximum risk for such an illness, usually of an affective nature. Worry concerning the fate of children can exacerbate the psychosis. Parents who have had a psychotic episode may need help in assessing and meeting their children's needs, both during and in the wake of the episode. In the longer term, since the children are at increased risk of psychiatric disorder for both genetic and environmental reasons, child psychiatry input may be required. Prevention, that is intervention to reduce the impact of disturbed parents on their children, may be better than cure.[260]

Accommodation

Moving house is a stressful event even for the most robust citizen, and the uncertainties around finding new accommodation can impair recovery in the psychotic patient. Therefore, wherever possible, young patients recovering from a first psychotic episode should return to their home with their parents or own family. However, should this not be possible, the services should be able to offer or obtain a range of accommodation, from hostels with intensive social and nursing support, to homes with a warden, to semi-independent and then totally independent living. Different patients may be able to progress through these stages of accommodation at different rates.

Day resource centres

It is important that the young patient should not be precipitously discharged from intensive support in hospital to a void in which he/she has no daily structure. If the young person is unable to return to study or work within a reasonably short period, then attendance at a resource centre may provide such a structure. Such a day programme should focus on recovery and learning new social or leisure skills or alternatively skills that will be useful in the workplace, for example computing. These programmes provide an invaluable opportunity to monitor progress and compliance with medication; indeed patients on once daily medication regimes can be given their medication at the centre. However, where possible, first-onset patients should not be invited to attend gloomy day centres largely inhabited by chronically unwell patients.

Self-help and support groups

These may also provide a valuable role in assisting in psychosocial adaptation, and patients and their families should be informed of the existence of such groups. The goals of these groups include:

- psychoeducation including destigmatization
- provision of fora for discussion
- advocacy
- influencing service provision
- working to achieve adequate support for treatment and research into mental illness

Alleviation of symptoms

Cognitive behavioural treatments (CBT) involving individual or group therapy are increasingly being used to alleviate psychotic symptoms. The use of CBT is based on the assumptions that (a) psychotic patients tend to employ dysfunctional cognitive models of themselves and others, and (b) these models are amenable to modification by psychological techniques.

The United Nations state that every person with a mental illness should have the right to live and work, as far as is possible, in the community.[261] In practice, however, the pervasive psychosocial sequelae of a first psychotic episode, in occupational, academic, financial, familial and social domains, may prevent the achievement of this ideal. To give a simple example, after a hospital admission for mania in the UK, driving is not allowed for 6 to 12 months by the Licensing Agency. A diagnosis of manic depression excludes patients from driving certain public service vehicles,[262] and may exclude patients from other occupations, depending on the attitude of the employer.

First episodes of psychosis often occur during late adolescence or early adult life when the affected individual is still in education or only beginning to establish their adult social and occupational role; the whole trajectory of their development may be impaired by a prolonged psychotic episode or its consequences. To prevent this, the clinician may need to liaise with the teacher, academic tutor or employer in order to provide appropriate information (with the patient's consent) and negotiate a graded return to study or work. If it does not seem feasible for the patient to return to their chosen field of study or work, a viable alternative should be explored. This may include the provision of sheltered work, or employment skills retraining. Setting of realistic and attainable short- and long-term goals may aid a sense of mastery and protect against a loss of self-esteem.[162] A vocational outcome should be a central aim of psychosocial interventions to facilitate recovery.[20]

Studies regarding social skills training in those suffering from chronic schizophrenia show a positive impact on behaviour, self-perception and social anxiety, with associated earlier hospital discharge and lower relapse rate.[263] Although there has been less work with first episode psychosis, the principles are equally applicable to certain patients, for example an adolescent with poor premorbid psychological and social adjustment. Social skills training involves the use of a wide range of techniques, including videotapes, modelling, role play, positive reinforcement and homework assignments, the content and style being tailored to the individual. Improvements in social adjustment may also be made via a group therapy approach for stable outpatients.[162]

The principles of cognitive behavioural therapy may be summarized as:

- identifying and measuring the target symptoms and behaviours

- examining their antecedents and consequences
- formulating, with the patient, more adaptive explanatory models for the targets
- evaluating the changes to target symptoms and behaviour

Mood disorder

Beck's cognitive therapy for depression has been adapted for use in bipolar affective disorder. The cognitive model of hypomania regards it as a mirror image of depression which is characterized by a positive cognitive triad of self, world and future, and positive cognitive distortions.[264] Positive cognitive distortions include:

- jumping to positive conclusions ('I'm a winner; I can do anything')
- underestimation of risk ('there's no danger here; I can surmount anything')
- minimization of problems ('nothing can go wrong')
- overvaluation of immediate gratification ('they should do what I want now')

The positive cognitive distortions provide reinforcing, biased confirmation of the positive cognitive triad. Positive experiences may be selectively attended to, and in this way underlying beliefs guiding behaviour are strengthened. Positive and negative schema are not mutually exclusive; an individual with a mixed affective episode may have both positive and negative (depressive) cognitive distortions.

Individual cognitive behavioural therapy for bipolar affective disorder includes the following components:[265]

- *assessment:* identification of core self-other schema and basic attitudes, triggering events, coping strategies and typical social behaviours (especially ways of perceiving and managing interpersonal conflict)
- *therapeutic work with the client:* aiming to provide psychoeducation regarding the nature of the disorder including the need to accept medication in a biopsychosocial view of the illness, insight into vulnerable self-other perceptions, strategies for challenging distortions in thinking, enhancement of constructive coping strategies (behavioural strategies) and early recognition of mood changes requiring preventative action

Delusions

The use of cognitive therapy for irrational beliefs was pioneered by Watts et al,[266] but it is only since the early 1990s that formal trials of its use in psychosis have been reported, particularly from psychologists in the UK. Cognitive therapy has been successfully used in the treatment of drug-refractory delusions,[267] and often includes elements of psychoeducation and compliance therapy, together with specific cognitive interventions targeted at the delusions. More recently, such CBT interventions have been applied to acute psychosis.[18,268]

This type of cognitive therapy may be successfully conducted in groups, together with psychoeducation.[18] Beliefs are challenged by other group members; 'facing up' to the illness rather than taking refuge in psychotic experiences is encouraged. Patients are empowered through identifying and exchanging helpful coping strategies for both negative and positive symptoms. Anxiety management including relaxation may also be taught.

Hallucinations

Psychological treatment aimed directly at auditory hallucinations is much less developed. It already shows promise, but its use in first-episode cases remains experimental. It should, therefore, generally be reserved for those first-episode cases in which auditory hallucinations fail to respond to more conventional therapy. Various options have been employed ranging from self-help groups to completing diaries on the monitoring of hallucinations. A number of recent approaches depend on the theory that auditory hallucinations represent a misperception of 'inner speech', and that consequently their content is important.[269]

Cognitive remediation

Recent years have seen a great expansion of neuropsychological research into schizophrenia, and elucidation of the deficits shown by patients.[270,271] Such deficits appear to have a more important impact on long-term social and occupational functioning than on clinical symptoms.[272] Some of the most important include:

- distractibility and attentional deficits
- memory problems
- limitations in planning and decision making

Remedial cognitive approaches are now being used as a means to ameliorate some of these. Cognitive remediation attempts to improve both clinical functioning and overall functioning by attempting to improve such neuropsychological deficits. The efficacy of individual cognitive remediation of the above deficits has been demonstrated in experimental trials,[273] but extended studies have not been carried out to correlate improvement in 'information processing under experimental conditions with measures of psychopathology or social functioning.[162]

In theory, cognitive remediation should ideally have a particular role in first-episode cases of schizophrenia with the hope that premorbid deficits might be improved and the development of further enduring cognitive deficits prevented.

The cognitive intervention focuses directly on the belief, the distress it causes, and the evidence for that belief, then invites the client to consider, in a collaborative manner, alternative constructions and meanings. Together with family engagement and a structured activity programme, this has been shown to result in a 25–50% reduction in time to recovery and a lower incidence of residual symptoms.[18] Cognitive-behavioural therapy has also been shown to be effective in the treatment of symptoms which have been resistant to medication for at least 6 months.[274]

Psychosocial approaches – 2
Enhancing recovery and
staying well

8

The clinician's responsibility does not end when his/her patient has recovered from the immediate crisis occasioned by their first psychotic episode. Indeed, one might say it is relatively easy to supervise such a recovery; it is more difficult to ensure that this lasts. In recent years, as the emphasis in psychiatry has switched to community care, a number of techniques have shown their value in preventing recurrence.

Case management

Before specialized techniques can be put into operation, it is necessary that the patient remains in contact with the services; too many patients do not do so, with resultant deterioration and eventual relapse. One technique which has been found to be valuable in facilitating continuity of care is case management. The principles are that immediately following recovery from the first episode:

- a care plan should be developed and agreed between the professional staff, patient and family
- a key worker should be designated whose responsibility it is to ensure that the patient receives the agreed care[275]

Enhancement of compliance with medication

Up to 50% of schizophrenic patients fail to comply with their treatment.[276,277] In one follow-up study of recent-onset manic patients, only 30% were found to be completely adhering to the treatment regime throughout the follow-up period.[278] Young patients who don't yet accept the fact, or the seriousness, of their illness are often particularly loath to continue to take medication after recovery from their first psychotic episode. Unfortunately, noncompliance results in high relapse and rehospitalization rates with significant cost not only the patient but also to carers and to the services.

Certain characteristics of patients are known to be associated with noncompliance. The risk factors for noncompliance in a first-episode psychosis include the following:[162,277,279–281]

- denial of illness
- cultural beliefs about illness (eg in minority groups)
- young age and male gender
- comorbid drug or alcohol abuse
- grandiose mood
- delusions (eg paranoid or regarding treatment)
- poor doctor–patient relationship
- misconceptions regarding treatment – fear of addiction, loss of control and loss of personality
- adverse effects of medication (previous or current)
- dislike of taking a substance which may control or alter mood
- dislike of the idea of chronic illness symbolized by a need for drug therapy

Drug-related beliefs are particularly important as they are often amenable to change, and patients who have a positive attitude to medication are more likely to be compliant even in the face of side-effects. This is not to say that the clinician should not do his/her utmost to avoid side-effects. Patients in their first episode of illness are often exquisitely sensitive to drugs, and once a patient has experienced, for example, an oculogyric crisis, the prospect of achieving a trusting therapeutic alliance is greatly diminished.

It is also important to recognize that patients' subjective experience of adverse effects of antipsychotics often differs from the view of the treating clinician. Both patients and clinicians notice EPS but while weight gain, memory disturbance, inability to concentrate and sexual problems are particularly disliked by those affected, other somatic side effects (eg tachycardia) may be more worrying to clinicians. Some studies suggest that subjective experience of adverse effects correlates better with compliance and quality of life than objective measures of adverse effects.[282]

Obviously, patients are more likely to comply with medication when drug treatment is seen as part of a wider package of care. Furthermore, didactic approaches have only a limited effect on noncompliance in patients with psychosis.[283] Better results are achieved when patients take an active role in monitoring their illness and decisions about treatment in a partnership with the clinician. Even the term 'noncompliance' may be inappropriate, implying a paternalistic clinician–patient relationship; a more acceptable term may be 'concordance' (referring to agreement between the views of the patient or their family and the clinician[285]). Methods of enhancing such concordance include an individual therapy approach with the patient, group therapy and family therapy.

Compliance therapy

Compliance therapy (CT) is a cognitive intervention which borrows principles from the technique of motivational interviewing,[284–286] and also uses insights gained from recent developments in cognitive behavioural therapy. Motivational interviewing aims to help people change their behaviour while avoiding the confrontation and stalemate of many conventional doctor–patient interactions.

Individual therapy

Compliance therapy is brief, pragmatic and eminently adaptable to a busy clinical setting. It may be given in four to six individual sessions, including the following components:[287]

- A review of the illness history, in order to formulate the patient's stance regarding the problem and treatment. If a patient denies that there is a problem, they may be asked why others think there is a problem, and how they evaluate similar behaviours in others, but if there is strong resistance to the notion of having a problem, then the issue is dropped. Basic information about psychotic symptoms is provided, aimed at decatastrophization, using normalizing rationale.[288]

- An exploration of ambivalence to treatment. The patient is asked to comment on common causes for resistance to treatment, which leads into a discussion of the patient's own misgivings regarding treatment, and the pros and cons of treatment.

- Treatment maintenance: stigma is combatted by reframing the use of medication as a freely chosen strategy to enhance quality of life. The prevalence of mental disorders is discussed, examples of famous sufferers are given, the analogy to physical illnesses such as diabetes is made and the patient's characteristic prodromal symptoms are identified in order to facilitate early intervention.

In a randomized controlled trial of compliance therapy (CT), at 18 months follow-up a significant reduction in the rehospitalization rate was found for the CT group (Figure 5).

Group and family therapy

The style and content of group or family therapy for compliance in psychosis has much in common with the individualized compliance therapy outlined above. Issues surrounding patients' ambivalence to medication are explored. A homogeneous group (for example all members suffering from a schizophrenia spectrum psychosis) may be more effective than a heterogeneous group, and those in later stages of recovery may assist in the educational process.[20] In family therapy, reasons for ambivalence including intrafamilial dynamic factors may be explored.[256]

Optimization of family attitudes and behaviour

The response of the family or other crucial individuals in the patient's immediate environment may influence the course of the illness, in terms of whether or not a recurrence of the psychosis occurs and the timing of recurrences. Evidence for this comes from a number of studies regarding the effect of high expressed emotion (EE) measure of the affective tone of relationships which consists of 3 separate attitudes:[289]

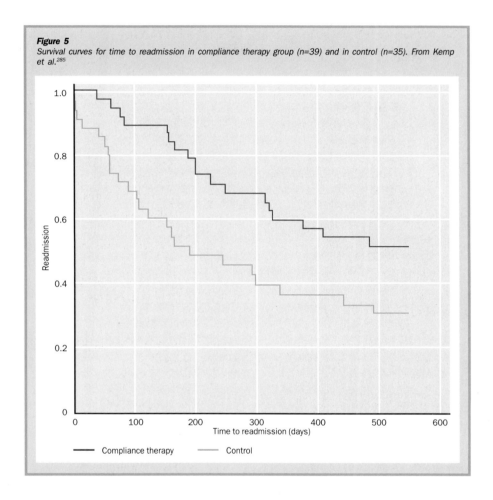

Figure 5
Survival curves for time to readmission in compliance therapy group (n=39) and in control (n=35). From Kemp et al.[285]

- criticism: statements of dislike, resentment, or annoyance, with accompanying negative voice tone

- hostility: statements indicating rejection of who the patient is as a person

- emotional overinvolvement: extremely protective, overconcerned, self-sacrificing attitudes regarding the patient.

Patients with both schizophrenia and bipolar illness have been found to relapse more frequently if they come from a high EE family than those from a low EE family;[278,290-292] however, interventions aimed at reducing EE may have less effect on relapse in patients with recent onset psychosis, possibly because of the fluid nature of family attitudes in this period.[293] There can be little doubt that diminution in the constant criticism that some patients receive from their families is likely to be beneficial, and in other cases a decrease of parental overinvolvement may allow the patient to assert his/her independence with resultant boosting of self-confidence. However, one should never blame family members; the relatives of psychotic patients often report distress, social isolation, and fears about their personal safety and financial consequences owing to assuming the carer role. Some families may prefer that the patient lives away from home, at least for a period. The provision of suitable alternative accommodation may then be necessary; if this involves the provision of a calm, structured environment, this may also benefit the patient.

Stress reduction

Other psychosocial stressors, or the patient's response to them, may be modifiable by psychotherapeutic avenues. There is evidence that stressful life events precipitate psychotic episodes.[102,294,295] Approaches such as interpersonal and rhythm stability therapy for bipolar affective disorder aim to provide a stress-buffering effect,[280] so that the risk of relapse in response to a stressor is reduced. This includes:

- daily ratings of mood, social, and circadian rhythms, to allow the patient to see the relationships between these and to identify environmental factors triggering disruption
- an 'interpersonal inventory' to identify interpersonal problem areas which may affect mood state and vice versa.

Promotion of early recognition of recurrence and appropriate intervention

The detection of early warning signs of an episode by an affected person or by others close to him/her may allow action to be taken to prevent escalation to frank psychosis. Each affected person tends to have their own specific early warning signs, or 'relapse signature'.[296] These may include the following:[257,278]

- *changes in affect*: suspiciousness, depression, anxiety and agitation, disinhibition with aggression or restlessness, feelings of tension, irritability, anger
- *changes in cognition*: odd ideas, vagueness, difficulties with concentration or recall
- *changes in beliefs or perceptions*: changes in view of self (especially with respect to others, eg ideas of reference, feeling superior to others or indispensible), of others or the world in general; perceptual abnormalities including alteration in perceived intensity of colours
- *physical changes*: sleep disturbance including atypical dreams, appetite change, somatic complaints, loss of energy or motivation, or increase in energy and activity

Many of the above are relatively nonspecific, it is the characteristic *constellation* of symptoms which comprises the 'relapse signature' for a particular individual.

Relapse prevention includes:

- adherence to medication
- avoidance of certain illicit drugs
- recognition of early warning signs
- psychosocial stress management
- effective help-seeking strategies
- maintaining a rewarding social or vocational role

Psychotherapeutic strategies for relapse prevention may be effectively conducted in a structured group setting,[256] and include the following components:

- discussion of specific relapse signatures
- daily record of mood state
- identification of situations which represent an increased risk of recurrence
- discussion of effect of relapse on self and others
- development of action plans should a recurrence occur

Family work may also be helpful for relapse prevention. Emphasis is put on seeing the family/friends/significant others as a vital part of the process of recovery and staying well. Each family member or other person with a significant relationship with the patient may be asked to separately list one major warning sign, following which these are compared and discussed. This may involve clarification of what does and what does not constitute 'danger signs', and what is illness and what is not.[256]

Support groups also advocate 'self-management' for relapse prevention, whereby a person takes increased responsibility for their own health.[297] This may include:

- developing skills of recognizing early warning signs
- strategies for appropriate action if early warning signs occur, including taking simple actions (eg exercise that the individual finds relaxing)
- self-medication: patients with good insight may be given a supply of medication and, through negotiation with their psychiatrist, adjust their dose of medication when early warning signs occur
- knowing triggers and taking preventative action if a known trigger is about to occur
- improving the quality of life: cultivating friends, having an interest or hobby, etc

Reduction of suicide risk

Patients recovering from a first psychotic episode are at a substantially increased risk of suicide, especially during the first

6 years.[33] If a suicide attempt occurs, chain analysis may be helpful,[298] whereby the sequence of events, behaviours, thoughts and interpersonal interchanges that precede and follow suicide attempts are clarified, and potentially more adaptive response patterns are explored with the patient.

Suicidal behaviour may be secondary to the lack of an alternative means of achieving valued goals and roles, the loss of social status, a sense of entrapment if psychotic relapses occur, or issues within the family.[19,280] Core problems of self-esteem and hopelessness are often underlying.[23]

In the particular context of a first episode of psychosis, one needs to establish whether the behaviour was driven by the psychotic experience as:

- a response to hallucinated commands
- an attempt to escape from continuously distressing psychotic experiences
- an attempt at self-sacrifice driven by delusions (eg to save the world)
- despair induced by the perception of irreparable damage done by the psychosis

In all cases, the behaviour should be treated with seriousness; in the first year after an episode of deliberate self-harm, there is a 1–2% risk of completed suicide, which is 100 times the general population risk.[299]

With the support of family members and significant others, the patient can be encouraged to communicate verbally the needs represented by the suicidal behaviour and to explore alternative problem-solving strategies in response to the stressors that precipitate these crises.

The question of 'insight-oriented' psychotherapy

Many of the above approaches could be said to be aimed at achieving a degree of personal growth. This can be further facilitated by means of personal therapy such as that developed by Hogarty and colleagues,[300] which uses behavioural techniques such as modelling, rehearsal, feedback and homework assignments; the efficacy of this approach has been demonstrated in controlled trials.

There is more controversy about 'insight-orientated' psychotherapy. Its advocates suggest that its addition may lead to:

- increased control over self-defeating behaviours
- emotional and interpersonal growth

Although exploratory psychotherapy has been advocated for psychosis,[301] much evidence indicates that intensive exploratory techniques during the acute phase of psychosis tend to prolong disorganization or precipitate relapse.[302] Very occasionally, exploratory therapy may, however, be indicated for a minority of patients, meeting the following criteria:[162]

- stable remission is achieved
- good therapeutic alliance is possible
- medication regimes are adhered to
- the capacity to tolerate and motivation to pursue insight-orientated work exist

Such an approach should be used very cautiously, and only when the patient him/herself is enthusiastically requesting it. It is important also that the patient's continuing progress should be closely monitored by an orthodox therapist while the exploratory therapy is being tried.

Course and outcome

The outlook for the person who presents with a first psychotic episode depends not only on the quality of the treatment they receive but also on the nature of the illness which gave rise to the initial breakdown. As the majority of first psychotic episodes are manifestations of either schizophrenia or bipolar affective disorder, one might think that the long-term outcome would be greatly influenced by which of these illnesses appears to underly the psychosis. However, as already discussed in Chapter 2, it can be difficult to make a reliable diagnosis in the first few months after the manifestation of psychotic symptoms. Furthermore, Van Os *et al*,[22] who followed-up a series of 166 recent-onset psychotic patients, found that description in terms of dimensions of psychosis was a better predictor of outcome than DSMIIIR diagnoses. Thus, those patients who showed an insidious onset and blunted affect tended to follow a chronic course while those patients who showed little insight had an outcome punctuated by compulsory admissions. The best outcome was found in those patients who had prominent affective symptoms, especially mania.

Two main kinds of investigations have examined the course and outcome of patients with their first episode of psychosis. The first type is the long-term retrospective study, often examining the patients' old medical files. The second is the prospectively designed cohort study. The latter provides more

reliable information but is far more difficult to conduct; first-episode patients are relatively few, and having recovered from what is almost invariably a deeply unpleasant experience, they are often difficult to maintain in follow-up. Nevertheless, it is possible, as shown by the study of Takei *et al*,[303] who followed up a series of patients who presented their first psychotic episode in 1973/4, and managed to trace more than 95% of subjects 18 years later; perhaps surprisingly, there was a high degree of concordance between the initial diagnosis and that at the 18-year follow-up.

Follow-up studies

A typical example of a prospective follow-up study is the 13-year study of a first-episode cohort identified in Nottingham by Mason *et al*;[304] the findings reported were similar to those from other long-term follow-up studies of schizophrenia.[305,306] In this study, 52% of patients were without psychotic symptoms over the last 2 years of follow up; however, 83% showed some degree of symptomatic or social disability, or continued in some form of psychiatric treatment or were dead. There is a general but unexplained finding that the outcome of psychosis appears to be better in developing rather than industrialized countries.[24,307]

A number of studies have looked at whether one can predict good or bad outcome for first episode or recent onset cases; recent examples of these include Lieberman *et al*[163] and Van Os *et al*.[22]

Predictors of favourable outcome

- good premorbid adjustment
- being married
- female sex
- having a sudden onset and florid psychotic presentation
- affective symptoms or a family history of affective illness
- obvious social precipitant
- living in a family with low 'expressed emotion'
- continued use of medication

Predictors of unfavourable outcome

- male sex and early onset
- a family history of schizophrenia
- longer duration of untreated illness
- structural brain abnormality on CT or MRI
- poor childhood social function
- low childhood IQ and/or educational achievement

The effect of duration of untreated illness on response to treatment is illustrated in Figure 6.

Neurodevelopmental abnormality

Numerous studies have shown that women experience a better post-illness course than men.[308–310] It has been suggested that this is because more male than female psychotic patients suffer from a neurodevelopmental disorder.[311] Indeed, it is clear that those other factors which are associated with a poor outcome are indicators of neurodevelopmental impairment, for example structural brain abnormalities or low childhood IQ.[312]

Employment

The best predictor of outcome is previous history.[313] High socio-economic background has also been found to be associated with a better chance of employment after the first psychotic episode.[314]

Social functioning

The evidence that the outcome of psychotic illness is more favourable in

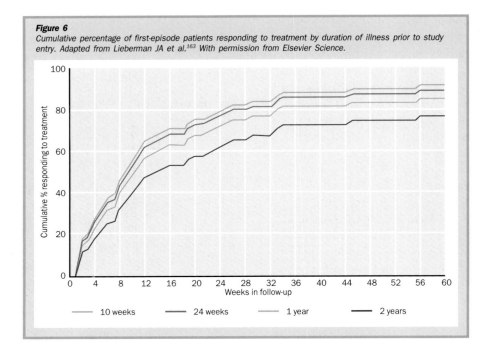

Figure 6
Cumulative percentage of first-episode patients responding to treatment by duration of illness prior to study entry. Adapted from Lieberman JA et al.[163] With permission from Elsevier Science.

developing than industrialized societies has prompted much interest in variations in sociocultural factors that might affect prognosis. It has been suggested that a higher level of social support and the presence of the extended family may contribute to this finding.[313] Having good social relationships appears to assist in the maintenance of mental health.[315–317]

Course of illness

Positive symptoms of schizophrenia tend to predominate in the earlier episodes of illness. During this period the disease tends to fluctuate and symptoms often respond well to treatment. Thus, the illness process appears to be most active at onset and early in its course, and the risk of rehospitalization is highest in the 5 years after first presentation; much of the deterioration takes place within the first 12–36 months. Relapses will not necessarily lead to further deterioration in the patient's condition and improvement may even occur in the very long term.[318] Some patients will experience further deterioration and possibly treatment resistance with each successive relapse. In general, it is thought that positive symptoms become less pronounced with time, while negative symptoms intensify.[319] Most readmissions occur in the first 5 years of illness, and between 10% and 40% of subjects never experience a readmission.[320]

There have been numerous studies in bipolar affective disorder attempting to identify predictors of course and outcome, but the findings have been inconsistent.[321,322]

After a first manic episode there is a high risk of early relapse, especially into depression, but psychosocial functioning appears to improve over time after recovery.[322]

The known predictors of favourable and unfavourable outcome may indicate that social and psychological factors influence how an individual handles their illness and at least in part determine the course and outcome. Psychosocial interventions could therefore affect the course and outcome by aiming to increase the number of favourable predictors for a given individual.

There is still much to be learnt in the area of first episode psychosis, with many studies currently being initiated. Our hope is that further information on all aspects of this important area will arise both from further research and from the application of new clinical approaches to those with their first episode of psychotic illness, and that with this, a course and outcome representing a significant improvement on that documented previously will be achieved.

References

1. Sullivan HS. The onset of schizophrenia, *Am J Psychiatry* 1927;**151(Suppl.6)**:135-139.

2. Cameron DE. Early Schizophrenia, *Am J Psychiatry* 1938;**95**:567-578.

3. Falloon IR. Early intervention for first episodes of schizophrenia: a preliminary exploration, *Psychiatry* 1992;**55(1)**:4-15.

4. Birchwood M, Macmillan F. Early intervention in schizophrenia, *Aust NZ J Psychiatry* 1993;**27(3)**:374-8.

5. Loebel AD, Lieberman JA, Alvir JM et al. Duration of psychosis and outcome in first-episode schizophrenia, *Am J Psychiatry* 1992;**149(9)**:1183-8.

6. Johnstone EC, Crow TJ, Johnson AL et al. The Northwick Park Study of first episodes of schizophrenia. I. Presentation of the illness and problems relating to admission, *Br J Psychiatry* 1986;**148**:115-20.

7. Beiser M, Erickson D, Fleming JA et al. Establishing the onset of psychotic illness, *Am J Psychiatry* 1993;**150(9)**:1349-54.

8. McGorry PD, Edwards J, Mihalopoulos C et al. EPPIC: an evolving system of early detection and optimal management, *Schizophr Bull* 1996;**22(2)**:305-26.

9. Hafner H, Maurer K, Loffler W et al. The influence of age and sex on the onset and early course of schizophrenia, *Br J Psychiatry* 1993;**162**:80-6.

10. Birchwood M, Cochrane R, MacMillan F et al. The influence of ethnicity and family structure on relapse in first-episode schizophrenia, *Br J Psychiatry* 1992;**161**:783-90.

11. McGorry PD, Singh B. Schizophrenia: risk and possibility of prevention. In: Raphael B and Burrows G, eds, *Handbook of Studies on Preventative Psychiatry*, The Netherlands: Elsevier Science, 1995, pp 491-514.

12. Waddington JL, Scully PJ, Youssef HA. Developmental trajectory and disease progression in schizophrenia: the conundrum, and insights from a 12-year prospective study in the Monaghan 101, *Schizophr Res* 1997;**23(2)**:107-18.

13. Wyatt RJ. Neuroleptics and the natural course of schizophrenia, *Schizophr Bull* 1991;**17(2)**:325-351.

14. Wyatt RJ. Early intervention for schizophrenia: can the course of the illness be altered? *Biol Psychiatry* 1995;**38(1)**:1-3.

15. Lincoln CV, McGorry PD. Who cares? Pathways to psychiatric care for young people experiencing a first episode of psychosis, *Psychiatric Services* 1996, Vol 46. No. 11. P. 1166-1171.

16. Dunn J, Fahy TA. Police admissions to a psychiatric hospital: demographic and clinical differences between ethnic groups, *Br J Psychiatry* 1990;**156** (special issue):373-8.

17. McEvoy JP, Hogarty GE, Steingard S. Optimal dose of neuroleptic in acute schizophrenia. A controlled study of the neuroleptic threshold and higher haloperidol dose, *Arch Gen Psychiatry* 1991;**48(8)**:739-45.

18. Drury V, Birchwood M, Cochrane R et al. Cognitive therapy and recovery from acute psychosis: a controlled trial (a) I. Impact on psychotic symptoms, *Br J Psychiatry* 1996;**169(5)**:593-601 and (b) II. Impact on recovery time, *Br J Psychiatry* 1996;**169(5)**:602-7.

19. Birchwood M, McGorry P, Jackson H. Early intervention in schizophrenia, *Br J Psychiatry* 1997;**170**:2-5.

20. McGorry PD, Edwards J. *Early Psychosis Training Pack*. Macclesfield, UK: Gardiner-Caldwell Communications Ltd, 1997.

21. Ram R, Bromet EJ, Eaton WW et al. The natural course of schizophrenia: a review of first-admission studies, *Schizophr Bull* 1992;**18(2)**:185-207.

22. Van Os J, Fahy T, Jones P et al.

Psychopathological syndromes in the functional psychoses: association with course and outcome. *Psychol Med* 1996;**26**:161-76.

23. Birchwood M, Mason R, MacMillan J et al. Depression, demoralisation and control over psychotic illness, *Psychol Med* 1993;**23**:387-395.

24. Thara R, Henrietta M, Joseph A et al. Ten-year course of schizophrenia-the Madras longitudinal study, *Acta Psychiatr Scand* 1994;**90(5)**:329-36.

25. Bleuler M. The long-term course of schizophrenia psychoses, *Psychol Med* 1974;**4**:244-54.

26. Carpenter WT Jr, Strauss JS. The prediction of outcome in schizophrenia. IV: Eleven-year follow-up of the Washington IPSS cohort, *J Nerv Ment Dis* 1991;**179(9)**:517-25.

27. Hafner H, Maurer K, Loffler W et al. The epidemiology of early schizo-phrenia. Influence of age and gender on onset and early course, *Br J Psychiatry* 1994;**Supplement (23)**:29-38.

28. Wing JK, Cooper JE, Sartorius N. *The Measurement and Classification of Psychiatric Symptoms* , Cambridge: Cambridge University Press, 1974.

29. Mullen PD. Mental states and states of mind. In: Murray RM, McGuthrie P, eds, *Essentials of Postgraduate Psychiatry*, 3rd edn (Cambridge University Press: Cambridge), 1997, pp 1-40.

30. The Maudsley Handbook of Practical Psychiatry. Goldberg D, ed, London:

Oxford University Press, 1997.

31. Van Os J, Marcelis M, Sham P et al. Psychopathological syndromes and familial morbid risk of psychosis, *Br J Psychiatry* 1997;**170**:241-6.

32. McPhillips MA, Kelly FJ, Barnes TR et al. Detecting comorbid substance misuse among people with schizophrenia in the community: a study comparing the results of questionnaires with analysis of hair and urine, *Schizophr Res* 1997;**25(2)**:141-8.

33. Westermeyer JF, Harrow M, Marengo JT. Risk for suicide in schizophrenia disorders, *J Nerv Ment Dis* 1991;**179**:259-69.

34. Van Os, Fahy T, Bebbington P et al. The influence of life events on the subsequent course and outcome of psychotic illness. A prospective follow up of the Camberwell Collaborative Psychosis Study, *Psychol Med* 1994;**24**:503-13.

35. Duggan CF, Sham P, Lee AS et al. Can future suicidal behaviour in depressed patients be predicted? *J Affect Disord* 1991;**22(3)**:111-8.

36. Castle D, Wessely SC, Van Os J, et al. *Psychosis in the inner city. The Camberwell first episode study*. Maudsley Monograph, 1998 (in press).

37. Foerster A, Lewis S, Owen M et al. Premorbid personality in psychosis: effects of sex and diagnosis, *Br J Psychiatry* 1991;**158**:171-6.

38. Foerster A, Lewis S, Owen M et al. Low birth-weight and a family history of schizophrenia predict poor premorbid functioning in psychosis, *Schizophr Res* 1991;**5**:3-20.

39. Cannon M, Jones P, Murray RM et al. Childhood laterality and later risk of schizophrenia in the 1946 British birth cohort, *Schizophr Res* 1997;**26**:117-120.

40. Walker EF, Grimes KE, Davis DM et al. Childhood precursors of schizophrenia: facial expressions of emotion, *Am J Psychiatry* 1993;**150(11)**:1654-60..

41. Jones P, Rodgers B, Murray R et al. Child development risk factors for adult schizophrenia in the British 1946 birth cohort, *Lancet* 1994;**344(8934)**:1398-402.

42. Davies NJ, Murray RM. Schizophrenia - A Neurodevelopmental or Neurodegenerative Disorder? In: Beninger R, Palomo T and Archer T, eds, *Strategies for Studying Brain Disorders 3. Dopamine Disease States*, Madrid: Editorra CYM, 1996, pp 537-553.

43. Done DJ, Crow TJ, Johnstone EC et al. Childhood antecedents of schizophrenia and affective illness: social adjustment at ages 7 and 11, *Br Med J* 1994;**309(6956)**:699-703.

44. Parnas J, Cannon TD, Jacobsen B et al. Lifetime DSM-III-R diagnostic outcomes in the offspring of schizophrenic mothers. Results from the Copenhagen High-Risk Study, *Arch Gen Psychiatry* 1993;**50(9)**:707-14.

45. Mednick SA, Mura E, Schulsinger F et al. Erratum and further analysis: (osm)perinatal conditions and infant development in children with schizophrenic parents(csm), *Soc Biol* 1973;**20(1)**:111-2.

46. Schulsinger F, Parnas J, Petersen ET et al. Cerebral ventricular size in the offspring of schizophrenic mothers. A preliminary study, *Arch Gen Psychiatry* 1984;**41(6)**:602-6.

47. Keith SJ, Matthews SM. The diagnosis of schizophrenia: a review of onset and duration issues, *Schizophr Bull* 1991;**17(1)**:51-67.

48. Fava GA, Kellner R. Prodromal symptoms in affective disorders, *Am J Psychiatry* 1991;**148(7)**:823-30.

49. Tennant CC. Stress and schizophrenia, *Integr Psychiatry* 1985;**3**:248-261.

50. Henderson AS. *An Introduction to Social Psychiatry*, Oxford: Oxford University Press, 1988.

51. Yung AR, McGorry PD. The prodromal phase of first-episode psychosis: past and current conceptualizations, *Schizophr Bull* 1996;**22(2)**:353-70.

52. Yung AR, McGorry PD, McFarlane CA et al. Monitoring and care of young people at incipient risk of psychosis, *Schizophr Bull* 1996;**22(2)**:283-303.

53. McGuffin P, Owen MJ, O'Donovan

MC et al. *Seminars in Psychiatric Genetics*. London: Royal College of Psychiatrists, Gaskell Press, 1994.

54. Sham PC, Jones P, Russell A et al. Age at onset, sex, and familial psychiatric morbidity: Report from the Camberwell Collaborative Psychosis Study, *Br J Psychiatry* 1994;**165**:466-73.

55. Gershon ES, Delisi LE, Hamovit J et al. A controlled family study of chronic psychoses. Schizophrenia and schizoaffective disorder, *Arch Gen Psychiatry* 1988;**45**:328-336.

56. Kendler KS, Diehl SR. The genetics of schizophrenia: a current, genetic-epidemiologic perspective, *Schizophrenia Bull* 1993;**19(2)**:261-285.

57. Baron M, Gruen R, Asius L et al. Schizoaffective illness, schizophrenia and affective disorders, morbidity risk and genetic transmission, *Acta Psychiatr Scand* 1982;**65**:253-262.

58. Bertelsen A, Harvald B, Hauge M. A Danish twin study of manic-depressive disorders, *Br J Psychiatry* 1977;**130**:330-351.

59. Heston LL. Psychiatric disorders in foster home reared children of schizophrenic mothers, *Br J Psychiatry* 1966;**112**:819-25.

60. Rosenthal D, Wender PH, Kety SS et al. Schizophrenics' offspring reared in adoptive homes. In: Rosenthal D and Kety SS, eds, *The Transmission of Schizophrenia*, Oxford: Pergamon Press, 1968.

61. Kendler KS, Gruenberg AM, Kinney DK. Independent diagnoses of adoptees and relatives as defined by DSM-II criteria, in the provincial and national samples of the Danish adoption study of schizophrenia, *Arch Gen Psychiatry* 1994;**51**:456-68.

62. Tienari P. Interaction between genetic vulnerability and family environment: the Finnish adoptive family study of schizophrenia, *Psychiatr Scand* 1991;**84(5)**:460-5.

63. Mendlewicz J, Rainer JD. Adoption study supporting genetic transmission in manic-depressive illness, *Nature* 1977;**268**:327-329.

64. Karayiorgou M, Gogos JA. Dissecting the genetic complexity of schizophrenia, *Mol Psychiatry* 1997;**2**:211-223.

65. Risch N, Botstein D. A manic depressive history, *Nat Genet* 1996;**12**:351-353.

66. Crocq M-A, Mant R, Asherson P et al. Association between schizophrenia and homozygosity at the dopamine D_3 receptor gene, *J Med Genet* 1992;**29**:858-860.

67. Shaikh S, Collier DA, Sham PC et al. Allelic association between a ser-9-gly polymorphism in the dopamine D_3 receptor gene and schizophrenia, *Hum Genet* 1996;**97**:714-19.

68. Williams J, Spurlock G, McGuffin P et al. Association between schizophrenia and T102C

polymorphism of the 5-hydroxytryptamine type 2a-receptor gene, *Lancet* 1996;**347**:1294-1296.

69. Nimgaonkar VL, Rudert WA, Zhang XR et al. Further evidence for association between schizophrenia the HLA DQB1 gene locus, *Schizophr Res* 1995;**18**:43-49.

70. Collier DA, Arranz MJ, Sham P et al. The serotonin transporter is a potential susceptibility factor for bipolar affective disorder, *NeuroReport* 1996;**7**:1675-1679.

71. Collier DA, Sham PC. Catch me if you can: are catechol and indolamine genes pleioptropic QTLs for common mental disorders? *Mol Psychiatry* 1997;**2**:181-183.

72. Carpenter NJ. Genetic anticipation. Expanding tandem repeats, *Neurol Clin* 1994;**12**:683-697.

73. O'Donovan MC, Guy C, Craddock N et al. Expanded CAG repeats in schizophrenia and bipolar disorder, *Nat Genet* 1995;**10**:380-381.

74. Morris AG, Gaitonde E, McKenna PJ et al. CAG repeat expansions and schizophrenia: assocation with disease in females and with early age-at-onset, *Hum Mol Genet* 1995;**4**:1957-61.

75. Cannon M, Jones P. Schizophrenia, *J Neurol Neurosurg Psychiatry* 1996;**61**:604-613.

76. McNeil TF, Cantor GE, Sjostrom K. Obstetric complications as antecedents of schizophrenia: Empirical effects of using different obstetric complication scales, *J Psychiatric Res* 1994;**28(6)**:519-30.

77. McGrath J, Murray RM. Risk factors for schizophrenia; from conception to birth. In: Hirsch S and Weinberger D, eds, *Schizophrenia*, Oxford: Blackwell, 1995, pp 187-205.

78. McNeil TF, Cantor GE, Nordstrom LG et al. Are reduced circumference at birth and increased obstetric complications associated only with schizophrenic psychosis? *Schizophr Res* 1996;**22**:41-47.

79. Kendell RE, Juszczak E, Cole SK. Obstetric complications and schizophrenia: A case control study based on standardised obstetric records, *Br J Psychiatry* 1996;**168(5)**:556-561.

80. Kunugi H, Takei N, Murray R M et al. Small head circumference at birth in schizophrenia, *Schizophr Res* 1996;**20**:165-170.

81. Verdoux H, Geddes J R, Takei N et al. Obstetric complications and age at onset in schizophrenia: an international collaborative meta-analysis of individual patient data, *Am J Psychiatry* 1997;**154**:1220-27.

82. Rifkin L, Lewis S, Jones PB et al. Low birth weight and schizophrenia, *Br J Psychiatry* 1994;**165**:357-362.

83. Hultman CM, Sparen P, Takei N et al. Prenatal and perinatal risk factors for schizophrenia, affective psychosis and reactive psychosis, *Br Med J* 1998; submitted for publication.

84. Bradbury TN, Miller GA. Season of birth in schizophrenia: a review of the evidence, methodology and etiology. *Psychol Bull* 1985;**98**:569-94.

85. Torrey EF, Miller J, Rawlings T et al. Seasonality of births in schizophrenia and bipolar disorder: a review of the literature. *Schizophr Res* 1997;**28**:1-38.

86. Isohanni M, Rantakallio P, Jones P et al. The predictors of schizophrenia in the 1966 Northern Finland birth cohort study. *Schizophr Res* 1997;**24**:251.

87. Woodruff PWR, Murray RM. The aetiology of brain abnormalities in schizophrenia. In: Ancill R, ed, *Schizophrenia: Exploring the Spectrum of Psychosis*, Chichester: Wiley & Sons: Chichester, 1994, pp 95-114.

88. Zipursky RB, Lim KO, Sullivan EV et al. Widespread cerebral gray matter volume deficits in schizophrenia, *Arch Gen Psychiatry* 1992;**49(3)**:195-205.

89. Harvey I, Ron M, du Barlay G et al. Reduction of cortical volume in schizophrenia on Magentic Resonance Imaging, *Psychol Med* 1993;**23**:591-604.

90. Bruton CJ, Crow TJ, Frith CD et al. Schizophrenia and the brain: A prospective clinico-neuropathological study, *Psychol Med* 1990;**20(2)**:285-304.

91. Fearon P, Cotter P, Murray RM (1997) Is the association between obstetric complications and schizophrenia mediated by glutamatergic excitotoxic damage in the foetal /neonatal brain? In: Reveley M and Deacon B, eds, *Psychopharmacology of Schizophrenia*, London: Chapman & Hall, 1998.

92. Weinberger DR. On the plausibility of the neurodevelopmental hypothesis of schizophrenia. A new understanding: neurobiological, *Neuropsychopharmacology* 1996;**14**: 15-115.

93. Murray RM, Lewis SW. Is schizophrenia a neurodevelopmental disorder? *Br Med J* 1987;**295**:681-682.

94. Mirsky AF, Silberman EK, Latz A et al. Adult outcomes of high-risk children: differential effects of town and kibbutz rearing, *Schizophr Bull* 1985;**11(1)**:150-4.

95. Cannon TD, Mednick SA, Parnas J et al. Developmental brain abnormalities inthe offspring of schizophrenic mothers. I. Contributions of genetic and perinatal factors, *Arch Gen Psychiatry* 1993;**50**:551-64.

96. Cannon TD. Abnormalities of brain structure and function in schizophrenia: implications for aetiology and pathophysiology, *Ann Med* 1996;**28**:533-9.

97. Kendler KS. Genetic epidemiology in psychiatry: taking both genes and

environment seriously, *Arch Gen Psychiatry* 1994;**52**:895-9.

98. Brown GW, Harris TO. *Social Origins of Depression: A Study of Psychiatric Disorder in Women*, London: Tavistock, 1978.

99. Bebbington P, Knipers E. Life events and social factors. In: Kavanagh DJ, ed, *Schizophrenia: An Overview and Practical Handbook*, London: Chapman & Hall, 1992, pp 126-44.

100. Ventura J, Nuechterlein KH, Lukoff D et al. A prospective study of stressful life events and schizophrenic relapse, *J Abnorm Psychol* 1989;**98(4)**:407-11.

101. Malla AK, Cortese L, Shaw TS et al. Life events and relapse in schizophrenia. A one year prospective study, *Soc Psychiatry Psychiatr Epidemiol* 1990;**25(4)**:221-4.

102. Bebbington PE, Wilkins S, Jones P et al. Life events and psychosis. Initial results from the Camberwell Collaborative Psychosis Study, *Br J Psychiatry* 1993;**162**:72-9.

103. Brown GW, Harris TO, Peto J. Life events and Psychiatric Disorders. Part 2: Nature of causal link, *Psychol Med* 1973;**3**:159-76.

104. Strakowski SM, Tohen M, Stoll AL et al. Comorbidty in psychosis at first hospitalisation, *Am J Psychiatry* 1993;**150(5)**:752-57.

105. Thornicroft G. Cannabis and psychosis. Is there epidemiological evidence for an association? *Br J Psychiatry* 1990;**157**:25-33.

106. Andreasson S, Allebeck P, Rydberg U. Schizophrenia in users and nonusers of cannabis. A longitudinal study in Stockholm County, *Acta Psychiatr Scand* 1989;**79(5)**:505-10.

107. Martinez-Arevalo MJ, Calcedo-Ordonez A, Varo-Prieto JR. Cannabis consumption as a prognostic factor in schizophrenia, *Br J Psychiatry* 1994;**164(5)**:679-81.

108. Linszen D et al. Cannabis abuse and the course of schizophrenic disorder, *Arch Gen Psychiatry* 1994;**51**:273-79.

109. McGuire PK, Jones P, Harvey I et al. Morbid risk of schizophrenia for relatives of patients with cannabis-associated psychosis, *Schizophr Res* 1995;**15(3)**:277-81.

110. Delay J, Deniker P, Harl J. Utilisation en therapeutique psychiatrique d'une phenothiazine d'action centrale elective, *Ann Med Psychol* 1952;112-7.

111. Kerwin RW. The new atypical antipsychotics. A lack of extrapyramidal side-effects and new routes in Schizophrenia Research, *Br J Psychiatry* 1994;**164**:141-8.

112. Lieberman JA. Atypical antipsychotic drugs as a first-line treatment of schizophrenia: a rationale and hypothesis, *J Clin Psychiatry* 1996;**57(suppl 11)**:68-71.

113. *British National Formulary, No 34*

(Sept 1997) London: British Medical Association, and Royal Pharmaceutical Society of Great Britain, 161–71.

114. Richelson E. Preclinical pharmacology of neuroleptics: focus on new generation compounds, *J Clin Psychiatry* 1996;**57(suppl 11)**:4–11.

115. Sodhi MS, Murray RM. Future therapies for schizophrenia, *Exp Opin Ther Patents* 1997;**7(2)**: 151–165.

116. Kopala LC, Kimberley PG, Honer WG. Extrapyrimmidal signs and clinical symptoms in first-episode schizophrenia: response to low-dose risperidone. *J Clin Psychopharmacol* 1997;**17**:308-312.

117. Seeman P, Lee T, Chau-Wong M et al. Antipsychotic drug doses and neuroleptic/dopamine receptors, *Nature* 1976;**261**:717-19.

118. Pilowsky LS, Costa DC, Ell PJ et al. Clozapine, single photon emission tomography, and the D_2 dopamine receptor blockade hypothesis of schizophrenia, *Lancet* 1992;**340**:199-202.

119. Farde L, Nordstrom AL, Wiesel FA. Positron emission tomographic analysis of central D_1 and D_2 dopamine receptor occupancy in patients treated with classical neuroleptics and clozapine. *Arch Gen Psychiatry* 1992;**49**:538-44.

120. Van Tol HHM, Bunzow JR, Guan HC et al. Cloning of the gene for human D_4 receptor with high affinity for the antipsychotic clozapine, *Nature* 1991;**350**:610-19.

121. Shaikh S, Collier DA, Sham P et al. Analysis of clozapine response and polymorphisms of the dopamine D_4 receptor gene (DRD4) in schizophrenic patients, *Am J Med Genet (Neuropsychiatric Genet)* 1995;**60**:??

122. Seeman P, Guan H-G, Van Tol HHM. Dopamine D_4 receptors elevated in schizophrenia, *Nature* 1993;**365**:441-445 (letter).

123. Okubo Y, Suhara T, Sudo Y et al. Possible role of dopamine D1 receptors in schizophrenia, *Mol Psychiatry* 1997;**2**:291-92.

124. Griffon N, Crocq M-A, Pilon C et al. Dopamine D_3 receptor gene: organization, transcript variants, and polymorphism associated with schizophrenia, *Am J Med Genet* 1996;**67(1)**:63-70.

125. Asherson P, Mant R, Holman S, et al. Linkage association and mutational analysis of the dopamine D3 receptor gene in schizophrenia. *Mol Psychiatry* 1996;**112**;125-32.

126. Pilowsky LS, Mulligan RS, Acton PD et al. Limbic selectivity of clozapine [letter], *Lancet* 1997;**350**:490-91.

127. Pilowsky LS, Busatto GR, Taylor M et al. *Dopamine D_2* receptor occupancy in vivo by the novel atypical antipsychotic olanzapine - a [123]IBZM single photon emission tomography

(SPET) study. *Psychopharmacology* 1996; **124**;148-43.

128. Weinberger DR, Lipska BK. Cortical maldevelopment, antipsychotic drugs and schizophrenia: a search for common ground. *Schizophrenia Res*;1995;**16(2)**;87-110.

129. Woodruff PWR, Phillips ML, Rushe T et al. Corpus callosum size and interhemispheric function in schizophrenia, *Schizophr Res* 1997;**23**:189-96.

130. Murray RM, Oon MCH, Smith A et al. A possible association between increased excretion of dimethyltryptamine and certain features of psychosis, *Arch Gen Psychiatry* 1979;**36**:644-49.

131. Arranz MJ, Collier DA, Sodhi MS et al. Association between clozapine response and allelic variation in the 5-HT$_{2A}$ receptor gene, *Lancet* 1995;**345**:281-82.

132. Sodhi MS, Arranz MJ, Curtis DA. Association between clozapine response and allelic variation in the 5-HT$_{2C}$ receptor gene, *NeuroReport* 1995;**7**:369-75.

133. Badri F, Masellis M, Petronis A. Dopamine and serotonin system genes may predict clinical response to clozapine, *Am J Hum Genet* 1996;**59(4)**:1423.

134. Debonnel G, Demontigny C. Modulation of NMDA and dopaminergic neurotransmissions by sigma ligands - possible implications for the treatment of psychiatric disorders, *Life Sci* 1996;**58(9)**:721-34.

135. Duinkerke SJ, Botter PA, Jansen AAI et al. Ritanserin, a selective 5-HT(2/1c) antagonist, and negative symptoms in schizophrenia: a placebo-controlled double-blind trial, *Br J Psychiatry* 1993;**163**:451-55.

136. Modell S, Naber D, Nolzbach R. Efficacy and safety of an opiate sigma-receptor antagonist (SL-82.0715|) in schizophrenic patients with negative symptoms - an open dose range study, *Pharmacopsychiatry* 1996;**29(2)**:63-66.

137. Dewey SL, Smith GS, Logan J et al. Serotonergic modulation of striatal dopamine measured with positron emission tomography (PET) and in vivo microdialysis, *J Neurosci* 1995;**15**:821-29.

138. Keks NA. Minimising the non-extrapyrimmidal side-effects of antipsychotics. *Acta Psychiatr Scand*;**94**;18-24.

139. Goldstein JM, Arvanitis LA. ICI 204,636 (Seroquel'): a dibenzothiazepine atypical antipsychotc. Review of preclinical pharmacology and highlights of phase II clinical trials, *CNS Drug Reviews* 1995;**1**:50-73.

140. Tollefson GD, Beasley Jr CM, Tran PV et al. Olanzapine versus haloperidol in the treatment of schizophrenia and schizoaffective and schizophreniform

disorders: results of an international collaborative trial, *Am J Psychiatry* 1997;**154**:457–65.

141. Van Kammen D, McEvoy JP, Targum SD. A randomized, controlled, dose-ranging trial of sertindole in patients with schizophrenia, *Psychopharmacology* 1996;**124**:168–75.

142. Marder SR, Meibach RC. Risperidone in the treatment of schizophrenia, *Am J Psychiatry* 1994;**151**:1825–35.

143. Saltz BL, Woener M, Kane JM et al Prospective study of tardive dyskinesia incidence in the elderly, *JAMA* 1991;**266**:2402–06.

144. Jeste DV, Caligiuri MP, Paulsen JS et al. Risk of tardive dyskinesia in older patients. A prospective longitudinal study of 266 outpatients, *Arch Gen Psychiatry* 1995;**52**:756–65.

145. Gerlach J, Lublin H, Peacock L. *Extrapyramidal symptoms during long-term treatment with antipsychotics*. Special focus on clozapine and D_1 and D_2 dopamine antagonists,*Neuropsychopharmacology*1996;**14(35)**:35S-39S.

146. Tooley PJH, Zuiderwijk P. Drug safety: exerience with risperidone.*Adv Therapy*1997;**14**:262-266.

147. Kane JM, Weinhold P, Kinon B et al. Prevalence of abnormal involunatary movements ('spontaneous

dyskinesias') in the normal elderly, *Psychopharmacol* 1982;**77**:105-08.

148. Steen VM, Lovlie R, MacEwan T, et al. Dopamine D_3-receptor gene variant and susceptibility to tardive dyskinesia in schizophrenic patients. *Mol Psychiatry* 1997; **2**:139-45.

149. Rossi A, Mancani F, Stratta P, et al. Risperidone, negative symptoms and cognitive deficit in schizophrenia : an open study. *Acta Psychiatr Scand*1997;**95**:40-43.

150. Zorn SH, Jones SB, Ward KM et al. Clozapine is a potent and selective muscarinic M_4 receptor agonist, *Eur J Pharmacol, Mol Pharmacol Section* 1994;**269**:R1-R2.

151. Fritze J, Elliger T. Pirenzepine for clozapine-induced hypersalivation, *Lancet* 1995; **346**:1034 (letter).

152. Szabadi E. Clozapine-induced hypersalivation, *Br J Psychiatry* 1997;**171**:89 (letter).

153. Ereshefsky L. Pharmacokinetics and drug interactions: update for new antipsychotics, *J Clin Psychiatry* 1996;**57(suppl 11)**:12-25.

154. Pilowsky LS, Ring H, Shrine PJ et al. Rapid tranquilisation, a survey of emergency prescribing in a general psychiatric hospital. *Br J Psychiatry*1992; **160**:831-5.

155. Nebert DW, McKinnon RA. Cytochrome P450: evolution and functional diversity, *Progr Liver Dis* 1994;**12**:63-97.

156. Andersson T. Pharmacokinetics,
metabolism and interactions of acid
pump inhibitors. Focus on
omeprazole, lansoprazole and
pantoprazole, *Clin Pharmacokinet*
1996;**31(1)**:9–28.

157. Dahl M-L, Bertilsson L. Genetically
variable metabolism of
antidepressants and neuroleptic drugs
in man, *Pharmacogenetics*
1993;**3**:61–70.

158. Daly AK, Brokmoller J, Broly F et al.
Nomenclature for human CYP2D6
alleles, *Pharmacogenetics*
1996;**6**:193–201.

159 Funderburg LG, Vertrees JE, True JE
et al. Seizure after the addition of
erythromycin to clozapine treatment,
Am J Psychiatry 1994;**151**:1840–41.

160. Hollister LE. Antipsychotic drugs. In:
Hollister LE, ed, *Clinical use of
psychotherapeutic drugs*, Springfield:
Charles C Thomas, 1973, pp13–55.

161. Crow TJ, Macmillan JF, Johnson AL
et al. The Northwick Park study of
first episodes of schizophrenia, II: a
randomised controlled trial of
prophylactic neuroleptic treatment,
Br J Psychiatry 1986;**148**:120–27.

162 American Psychiatric Association
practice guidelines. Work group on
schizophrenia. Practice Guideline for
the treatment of patients with
schizophrenia, *Am J Psychiatry*1997;
154, vol 4. (April suppl): 1–63.

163. Lieberman JA, Alvir JM, Koreen A et
al. Psychobiologic correlates of
treatment response in schizophrenia,
Neuropsychopharmacology,
1996;**14(3S)**:13S–21S.

164. Atkin KA , Kendall F, Gould D et al.
Neutropenia and agranulocytosis in
patients receiving clozapine in the
UK and Ireland, *Br J Psychiatry*
1996;**169**:483–88.

165. May PR, Tumka AH, Yale C et al.
Schizophrenia: a follow-up study of
results of treatment. II: hospital stay
over 2 or 5 years, *Arch Gen
Psychiatry* 1976;**1976**:481-86.

166. Gallhofer B. First episode
schizophrenia: the importance of
compliance and preserving cognitive
function, *J Practical Psychiatry and
Behav Health* 1996;**2(2, suppl)**:
16S–24S.

167. Fulton B, Goa KL. Olanzapine. A
review of its pharmacological
properties and therapeutic efficacy in
the management of schizophrenia
and related psychoses, *Drugs*
1997;**53(2)**:81–298.

168. Nyberg S, Nordstrom CH, Farde L.
Positron emission tomography studies
on D2 dopamine receptor occupancy
and plasma antipsychotic levels in
man.*Int Clin Psychopharm*1995;
10;81–5.

169. Peuskens J, on behalf of the
Risperidone Study Group.
Risperidone in the treatment of
patients with chronic schizophrenia:
a multi-national, multi-centre, double-
blind, parallel-group study versus

haloperidol, *Br J Psychiatry* 1995;**166**:712-26.

170. Aitchison KJ, Kerwin RW. Cost-effectiveness of clozapine. A UK clinic-based study, *Br J Psychiatry* 1997;**171**: 125-30.

171. Guest JF, Hart WM, Cookson RF, et al. Pharmacoeconomic evaluation of long term treatment with risperidone for patients with schizophrenia .*Br J Med Econ*1996; **10**;59-67.

172. Albright PS, Livingstone S, Keegan DL, et al. Reduction of healthcare resource utilisation and costs following the use of risperidone for patients with schizophrenia previously treated with standard antipsychotic therapy. *Clin Drug Invest*1996;**11**;289-299.

173. Van Putten T, Marder SR, May PRA et al. Plasma levels of haloperidol and clinical response, *Psychopharmacol Bull* 1985;**21**:69-72.

174. Wode-Helgodt B, Borg S, Fyro B et al. Clinical effects and drug concentrations in plasma and cerebrospinal fluid in psychotic patients treated with fixed doses of chlorpromazine, *Acta Psychiatr Scand* 1978;**58**:149-73.

175. Baldessarini RJ, Cohen BM, Teicher MH. Significance of neuroleptic dose and plasma level in the pharma-cological treatment of psychoses, *Arch Gen Psychiatry* 1988;**45**:79-90.

176. Schooler et al (1997). Personal communication.

177. Wolkin A, Barouch F, Wolfe AP. Dopamine receptor blockade and clinical response: evidence for two biological subgroups of schizophrenia, *Am J Psychiatry* 1989;**146**:905-08.

178. Thompson C. The use of high dose antipsychotic medication. *Br J Psychiatry*1994;**164**;448-58.

179. Gill M, Hawi A, Webb M. *Homozygous mutation at cytochrome P4502D6 in an individual with schizophrenia: implications for antipsychotic drugs, side effects and compliance, Ir J Psych Med* 1997; **14(1)**:38-9.

180. Birchwood M, Todd P, Jackson C. Early intervention in psychosis; the critical period hypothesis.*Int Clin Psychopharmacol*1997;**12(8)**;S29-S38.

181. Davis JM. Overview: maintenance therapy in psychiatry, I: schizophrenia, *Am J Psychiatry* 1975;**132**:1237-45.

182. Kane JM. Treatment programme and long-term outcome in chronic schizophrenia, *Acta Psychiatr Scan* 1990;**(Suppl) 358**:151-57.

183. Bollini P, Pampollona S, Orza MJ et al. Antipsychotic drugs: is more worse? A meta-analysis of the published randomized controlled trials, *Psychol Med* 1994;**24**:307-16.

184. Kissling W (ed). *Guidelines for Neuroleptic Relapse Prevention in Schizophrenia*, Berlin: Springer-Verlag: Berlin, 1991.

185. Carpenter WT Jr, Heinrichs DW,

Hanlon TE. A comparative trial of pharmacologic strategies in schizophrenia, *Am J Psychiatry* 1987;**144**:1466-70.

186. Herz MI, Glazer WM, Mostert MA et al. Intermittent vs maintenance medication in schizophrenia: two-year results, *Arch Gen Psychiatry* 1991;**48**:333-39.

187. Jolley AG, Hirsch SR, McRink A et al. Trial of brief intermittent neuroleptic prophylaxis for selected schizophrenic outpatients: clinical outcome at one year, *Br Med J* 1989;**298**:985-90.

188. Gaebel W. Is intermittent early intervention medication an alternative for neuroleptic maintenance treatment? *Int Clin Psychopharmacol* 1995;**9**:11-16.

189. Davis JM, Janicak P, Singla A et al. Maintenance antipsychotic medication. In: Barnes TRE, ed, *Antipsychotic Drugs and their Side Effects*, London: Acdemic Press, 1993, pp183-203.

190. Gerlach J. Depot neurolptics in relapse prevention: advantages and disadvantages, *Int Clin Psychopharmacol* 1995;**9**:12-20.

191. Barnes TRE. Clinical assessment of the extrapyramidal side effects of antipsychotic drugs, *J Psychopharmacol* 1992;**6(2)**:214-21.

192. Van Putten T. Why do schizophrenic patients refuse to take their drugs? *Arch Gen Psychiatry* 1974;**31**:67-72.

193. Drake RE, Ehrlich J. Suicide attempts associated with akathisia, *Am J Psychiatry* 1985;**142**:499-501.

194. Casey DE. Side effect profiles of new antipsychotic agents, *J Clin, Psychiatry* 1996;**57(suppl 11)**:40-45.

195. Szabadi E. Adverse reactions profile:11 Antipsychotic drugs, *Prescribers' Journal* 1995;**35(1)**:37-44.

196. Keck PI Jr, Pope HG Jr, McElroy SL. Frequency and presentation of neuroleptic malignant syndrome: a prospective study, *Am J Psychiatry* 1987;**144**:1344-46.

197. Mandel A, Gross M. Agranulocytosis and phenothiazines, *Dis Nerv System* 1986;**29**:32-36.

198. Kane J, Honigfeld G, Singer J et al. Clozapine for the treatment-resistant schizophrenic: a double-blind comparison with chlorpromazine, *Arch Gen Psychiatry* 1988;**45**:789-96.

199. Burke RE, Fahn S, Jankovic J et al. Tardive dystonia: late-onset and persistent dystonia caused by antipsychotic drugs, *Neurol* 1982;**32**:1335-46.

200. Van Os J, Fahy T, Jones P et al. Tardive dyskinesia: who is at risk? *Acta Psychiatr Scan* 1997;**96**:206-16.

201. Waddington JL. Psychopathological and cognitive correlates of tardive dyskinesia in schizophrenia and other disorders treated with neuroleptic drugs, *Adv Neurol* 1995;**65**:211-29.

202. Lieberman JA, Saltz BL, Johns CA et al. The effects of clozapine on tardive dyskinesia, *Br J Psychiatry* 1991;**158**:503-10.

203. Prien RF, Caffey EM, Klett CJ. Comparison of lithium carbonate and chlorpromazine in the treatment of mania. Report of the Veterans Administration and National Institute of Mental Health Collaborative Study Group, *Arch Gen Psychiatry* 1972;**26**:146-53.

204. Lingjaerde O, Ahlfors UG, Bech P et al. The UKU side effect rating scale: a new comprehensive rating scale for psychotropic drugs and a cross-sectional study of side effects in neuroleptic-treated patients, *Acta Psychiatrica Scan* 1987;**76(suppl 334)**:100.

205. Sachs GS. Bipolar mood disorder: practical strategies for acute and maintenance phase treatment, *J Clin Psychopharmacol* 1996;**16(2)**:32S-47S.

206. Chouinard G. Clonazepam in acute and maintenance treatment of bipolar affective disorder, *J Clin Psychiatry* 1987;**48(10, suppl)**:29-36.

207. Bradwejn J, Shriqui C, Koszycki D et al. Double-blind comparison of the effect of clonazepam and lorazepam in acute mania, *J Clin Psychopharmacol* 1990;**10**:403-8.

208. Lenox RH, Newhouse PA, Creelman WL et al. Adjunctive treatment of manic agitation with lorazepam versus haloperidol: a double blind study. *J Clin Psychiatry* 1992;**53(2)**:47-52.

209. Montgomery SA. Selective serotonin reuptake inhibitors in the acute treatment of depression. In: Bloom FE, Kupfer DJ, ed, *Psychopharmacology: the Fourth Generation of Progress*, New York: Raven Press, 1995, pp 1043-51.

210. Goodwin FK, Jamison KR. *Manic-Depressive Illness*, New York: Oxford University Press, 1990.

211. Cohen WJ, Cohen NH. Lithium carbonate, haloperidol, and irreversible brain damage, *JAMA* 1974;**230**:1283-87.

212 Loudon JB, Waring H. Toxic reactions to lithium and haloperidol [letter], *Lancet* 1976;**2**:1088.

213. Johnson DAW, Lowe MR, Barchelor DH. Combined lithium-neuroleptic therapy for manic-depressive illness, *Hum Psychopharmacol* 1990;**5(suppl)**:262-97.

214. Cookson J. Lithium and other drug treatments for recurrent affective disorder. In: Checkley SA, ed, *The Management of Depressive Illness*, Oxford: Blackwell Science, (in press).

215. Rasmussen J, Hallstrom C. What drugs can do to help. In: Varma V, ed, *Managing Manic Depressive Disorders*. London: Jessica Kingsley, 1997.

216. Klawans HL, Wiener WJ. The pharmacology of choreatic movements, *Progr Neurobiol* 1976;**6(1)**:49-80.

217. McElroy SK, Keck PE et al. Valproate

in the treatment of acute mania: a placebo-controlled study, *Arch Gen Psychiatry* 1991;**48**:62-68.

218. Bowden CL, Brugger AM, Swann AC et al. Efficacy of divalproex vs lithium and placebo in the treatment of mania, *JAMA* 1994;**271**:918-24.

219. Freeman TW, Clothier JL, Passagil P et al. A double-blind comparison of VPA and lithium in the treatment of acute mania, *Am J Psychiatry* 1992;**149**:108-11.

220. Calabrese JR, Woyshville MJ, Kinnel SE et al. Mixed states and bipolar rapid cycling and their treatment with VPA, *Psychiatr Ann* 1993;**23**:70-78.

221. Keck PE Jr, McElroy SL, Tugrul KC et al. Valproate oral loading in the treatment of acute mania, *J Clin Psychiatry* 1993;**54**:305-8.

222. Maes M, Calabres JR. Mechanisms of action of valproate in affective disorders. In: Joffe RT and Calabrese JR, eds, *Anti-convulsants in Mood Disorder*, New York: Marcel Dekker, 1994, pp 93-110.

223. Post RM, Denicoff KD, Frye MA et al. Re-evaluating carbamazepine prophylaxis in bipolar disorder, *Br J Psychiatry* 1997;**170**:202-04.

224. Placidi GF, Lenzi A, Lazzerine F et al. The comparative efficacy and safety of carbamazepine versus lithium: a randomized, double-blind 3-year trial in 83 patients, *J Clin Psychiatry* 1986;**47**:490-4.

225. Schubert T, Stoll I, Miller WE. Therapeutic concentrations of lithium and carbamazepine inhibit cGMP accumulation in human lymphocytes: a clinical model for possible common mechanism of action? *Psychopharmacology* 1991;**104**:45-50.

226 Weiss SRB et al. Cross-tolerance between carbamazepine and valproate in an amygdala kindled seizure paradigm, *Soc Neurosci Abstracts* 1991;**6**:1256.

227. Zis AP, Grof P, Webster M et al. The cyclicity of affective disorders and its modification by drugs, *Psychopharmacol* 1980;**16**:47-9.

228. Angst J. Course of affective disorders. In: Van Praag HM, Lader HM, Rafaelson OJ et al, eds, *Handbook of Biological Psychiatry*, New York: Marcel Dekker, 1981, pp 225-42.

229. Guscott R, Taylor L. Lithium prophylaxis in recurrent affective illness. Efficacy, effectiveness, and efficiency, *Br J Psychiatry* 1994;**164**:741-46.

230. Moncrieff J. Lithium: evidence reconsidered, *Br J Psychiatry* 1997;**171**:113-19.

231. Cookson J. Lithium: balancing risks and benefits, *Br J Psychiatry* 1997;**171**:120-24.

232. Goodwin GM. Recurrence of mania after lithium withdrawal. Implications for the use of lithium in the treatment of bipolar affective

disorder, *Br J Psychiatry*
1994;**164**:149-52.

233. Baldessarini RJ, Tondo L, Faedda GL
et al. Effects of the rate of
discontinuing lithium maintenance
treatment in bipolar disorders, *J Clin
Psychiatry* 1996;**57**:441-48.

234. Faedda GL, Tondo L, Baldessarini RJ
et al. Outcome after rapid vs gradual
discontinuation of lithium treatment
in bipolar mood disorders, *Arch Gen
Psychiatry* 1993;**50**:448-55.

235. Baldessarini RJ, Tondon L, Floris G et
al. Reduced morbidity after gradual
discontinuation of lithium treatment
for bipolar I and II disorders: a
replication study, *Am J Psychiatry*
1997;**154(4)**:551-53.

236. Mander AJ. Is there a lithium
withdrawal syndrome? *Br J
Psychiatry* 1986;**149**:598-01.

237. Paselow Ed, Fieve RR, Di Faglia, et al.
Lithium prophylaxis of bipolar illness:
the value of combination
treatment.*Br J Psychiatry*
1994;**164**:208-14.

238. O'Connell RA, May JA, Flatow L et al.
Outcome of bipolar disorder on
longterm treatment with lithium, *Br J
Psychiatry* 1991;**159**:123-129.

239. Prien RF, Kupfer DJ, Mansky PA et
al. Drug therapy in the prevention of
recurrences in unipolar and bipolar
affective disorder: Report of the
NIMH Collaborative Study Group
comparing lithium carbonate,
imipramine, and a lithium carbonate -

imipramine combination, *Arch Gen
Psychiatry* 1984;**41**:1096-1104.

240. McElroy SL, Pope HG Jr, Keck PE Jr
et al. Treatment of psychiatric
disorders with sodium valproate: a
series of 73 cases, *Psychiatrie
Psychobiologie* 1988;**3**:81-5.

241. Lambert PA and Venaud G.
Comparative study of valpromide
versus lithium in the treatment of
affective disorders, *Nervure*
1992;**5(2)**:57

242. Bowden CL. *Maintenance strategies
for bipolar disorder*. Presented at
American Psychiatric Association
Congress New York, May 1996.

243. Gelenberg AJ, Kane JM, Keller MB et
al. Comparison of standard and low
serum levels of lithium for
maintenance treatment of bipolar
disorder, *N Eng J Med*
1989;**321**:1489-1493.

244. McElroy SL, Keck PE, Pope HG et al.
Valproate in the treatment of bipolar
disorder: literature review and
clinical guidelines, *J Clin Pharmacol*
1992;**12**:42S-52S.

245. Taylor D, Duncan D. Doses of
carbamazepine and valproate in
bipolar affective disorder, *Psychiatric
Bull* 1997;**21**:221-223.

246. Schou M. *Lithium Treatment of
Manic-depressive Illness: A Practical
Guide*, Basel: Karger, 1993.

247. Waller D. Lithium-induced polyuria,
Prescribers' Journal
1997;**37(1)**:24-28.

248. Schou M. Artistic productivity and lithium prophylaxis in manic-depressive illness, *Br J Psychiatry* 1979;**135**:97-103.

249. Levy RH and Penry JK, eds, *Idiosyncratic reactions to valproate: clinical risk patterns and mechanisms of toxicity*, New York: Raven Press, pp 1099-111.

250. Green RS. Why schizophrenic patients should be told their diagnosis, *Hosp Comm Psychiatry* 1984;**35**:76-7.

251. Hogarty GE. Prevention of relapse in chronic schizophrenic patients, *J Clin Psychiatry* 1993;**54**:18-23.

252. Nayani TH, David AS. The auditory hallucination: a phenomenological survey, *Psychol Med* 1996;**26**:177-189.

253. Taylor S. Adjustment to threatening events: a theory of cognitive adaptation, *Psychologist* 1983;**38**:1161-1173.

254. McGorry PD. Psychoeducation in first-episode psychosis: a therapeutic process, *Psychiatry* 1995;**58**:313-327.

255. Yalom ID. *The Theory and Practice of Group Psychotherapy*, 3rd ed, New York: Basic Books, 1985.

256. Asen EK. What relatives and friends can do to help. In: Varma V, ed, *Managing Manic Depressive Disorders*, London: Jessica Kingsley, 1997.

257. Miklowitz DJ, Goldstein MJ. Behavioural family treatment for patients with bipolar affective disorder, *Behav Modif* 1990;**14**:457-489.

258. Kellam SG, Goldberg SC, Schooler NR et al. Ward atmosphere and outcome of treatment of acute schizophrenia, *J Psychiatr Res* 1967;**5**:145-63.

259. Raskis H. Cognitive restructuring: why research is therapy, *Arch Gen Psychiatry* 1960;**2**:612-21.

260. Cowling VR, McGorry PD, Hay DA. Children of parents with psychotic disorders, *Med J Aust* 1995; **163**: 119-120.

261. United Nations Principles for the protection of persons with mental illness and the improvement of mental healthcare, 1990, adopted by General Assembly resolution 46/119.

262. Cookson JC. Manic-depressive illness and driving, *Travel Med International* 1989;**7**:105-108.

263. Benton MK, Schroeder HE. Social skills training with schizophrenics: a meta-analytic evaluation, *J Consult Clin Psychol* 1990;**58(6)**:741-47.

264. Newman C, Beck AT. *Cognitive Therapy of Rapid Cycling Bipolar Affective Disorder - Treatment Manual*. Philadelphia: Centre for Cognitive Therapy, University of Pennsylvania, 1993.

265. Palmer A, Gilbert P. What psychologists can do to help. In: Varma V, ed, *Managing Manic Depressive Disorders*, London: Jessica Kingsley, 1997.

266. Watts FN, Powell GE, Austin SV. The modification of abnormal beliefs, *Br J Med Psychol* 1973;**46**:359–363.

267. Garety PA, Kuipers L, Fowler D et al. Cognitive behaviour therapy of schizophrenia, *Br J Med Psychol* 1994;**67**:259–271.

268. Jackson H, McGorry PD, Edwards J et al. Cognitively-oriented psychotherapy for early psychosis (COPE). In: Cotton PJ, and Jackson J, eds, *Early Intervention and Preventative Application of Clinical Psychology*, Melbourne: Academic Press, 1997.

269. Cahill C, Silbersweig D, Frith C. Psychotic experience in deluded patients using distorted auditory feedback. *Cognitive Neuropsychiatry* 1997;**1**;201–3.

270. Saykin AJ, Shtasel DL, Gur RE et al. Neuropsychological deficits in neuroleptic naive patients with first-episode schizophrenia, *Arch Gen Psychiatry* 1994;**51(2)**:124–31.

271. Morris RG, Rushe T, Woodruff PW et al. Problem solving in schizophrenia: a specific deficit in planning ability, *Schizophr Res* 1995;**14(3)**:135–46.

272. Green MF. Cognitive remediation in schizophrenia: is it time yet? *Am J Psychiatry* 1993;**150**:178–187.

273. Corrigan PW, Yodufsky SC (eds). *Cognitive Remediation for Schizophrenia* Washington DC: American Psychiatric Press, 1994.

274. Kuipers E, Garety P, Fowler D et al. London-East Anglia randomised controlled trial of cognitive-behavioural therapy for psychosis, *Br J Psychiatry* 1997;**171**:319–327.

275. Creed F et al (on behalf of the UK 700 group). Case management, *Br J Psychiatr*, submitted.

276. Corrigan PW, Liberman RP, Engel JD. From non-compliance to collaboration in the treatment of schizophrenia, *Hosp Comm Psychiatry* 1990;**41**:1203–1211.

277. Bebbington PE. The content and context of compliance, *Int Clin Psychopharmacol* 1995;**9**:41–50.

278. Miklowitz DJ, Goldstein MJ, Nuechterlein KH, et al. Family factors and the course of bipolar affective disorder. *Arch Gen Psychiatry* 1988;**45**:225–31.

279. Goldstein MJ. Psychosocial strategies for maximizing the effects of psychotropic medications for schizophrenia and mood disorder, *Psychopharmacol Bull* 1992;**28**:237–240.

280. Miklowitz DJ. Psychotherapy in combination with drug treatment for bipolar disorder, *J Clin Psychopharmacol* 1996;**16(2, suppl 1)**:56S–66S.

281. Jamison KR, Gerner RH, Goodwin FK. Patient and physician attitudes toward lithium: relationship to compliance, *Arch Gen Psychiatry* 1979;**36**:866–9.

282. Naber D. A self-rating to measure

subjective effects of neuroleptic
drugs, relationships to objective
psychopathology, quality of life,
compliance and other clinical
variables, *Int Clin Psychopharmacol*
1995;**10 (suppl 3)**:133–138.

283. Kemp R, Hayward P, Applethwaite G
et al. Compliance therapy in psychotic
patients: a randomised controlled trial,
Br Med J 1996;**312**:345–349.

284. Kemp R, Kirov G, Everitt B et al. A
randomised controlled trial of
compliance therapy: 18-month
follow-up, *Br J Psychiatry* (in press).

285. Mullen PD. Compliance becomes
concordance. Making a change in
terminology produces a change in
behaviour, *Br Med J*
1997;**314**:691–692.

286. Rollnick S, Heather N, Bell A.
Negotiating behaviour change in
medical settings. The development of
brief motivational interviewing, *J
Mental Health UK* 1992;**1(1)**:25–37.

287. Kemp R, David A. Compliance
therapy: an intervention targeting
insight and treatment adherence in
psychotic patients, *Behav Cogn
Psychotherapy* 1996;**24**:331–350.

288. Kingdon DG, Turkington D.
*Cognitive-Behavioural Therapy of
Schizophrenia*, New York: Guildford
Press, 1994.

289. Vaughn CE, Leff JP. The influence of
family and social factors on the
course of psychiatric illness, *Br J
Psychiatry* 1976;**148**:642–7.

290. Lam DH. Psychosocial family
intervention in schizophrenia: a
review of empirical studies, *Psychol
Med* 1991;**21**:423–441.

291. Kuipers L, Birchwood M, McCreadie
RG. Psychosocial family intervention
in schizophrenia: a review of
empirical studies, *Br J Psychiatry*
1992;**160**:272.

292. Tarrier N, Barrowclough C, Vaughn C
et al. The community management of
schizophrenia: a controlled trial of
behavioural intervention with families
to reduce relapse, *Br J Psychiatry*
1988;**153**:532–542.

293. Linszen D, Dingemans P, van der
Does JW et al. Treatment, expressed
emotion, and relapse in recent onset
schizophrenic disorders, *Psychol Med*
1996;**26**:333–342.

294. Day R, Nielsen H, Korton A et al.
Stressful life events preceding the
acute onset of schizophrenia: a cross-
national study from the World Health
Organization, *Culture Med
Psychiatry* 1987;**11**:1–123.

295. Johnson SL, Roberts JE. Life events
and bipolar disorder: implications
from biological theories, *Psychol Bull*
1995;**117**:434–49.

296. Smith JA, Tarrier N. Prodromal
symptoms in manic depressive
psychosis, *Soc Psychiatry Psychiatr
Epidemiol* 1992;**27(5)**:245–248.

297. Guiness D. A guide to self-
management. In: Varma V, ed,
Managing Manic Depressive

Disorders, London: Jessica Kingsley, 1997.

298. Linehan M. *Cognitive-behavioural Treatment of Borderline Personality Disorder*, New York: Guildford Press, 1993.

299. Kreitman N (ed). *Parasuicide*, London: J Wiley, 1977.

300. Hogarty GE, Kornblith SJ, Greenwald D et al. Personal therapy: a disorder-relevant psychotherapy for schizophrenia, *Schizophr Bull* 1995;**21(3)**:379-93.

301. Jackson M, Williams P. *Unimaginable Storms*, London: H Karnac, 1994.

302. Mueser KT, Berenbaum H. Psychodynamic treatment of schizophrenia: is there a future? *Psychol Med* 1990;**20**:253–262.

303. Takei N, Persaud R, Woodruff et al. Eighteen year follow-up of Afro–Caribbean and white patients with their first episode of psychosis: a population-based study, *Br J Psychiatry* 1998 (in press).

304. Mason P, Harrison G, Glazebrook C et al. Characteristics of outcome in schizophrenia at 13 years, *Br J Psychiatry* 1995;**167(5)**:596-603.

305. The Scottish Schizophrenia Research Group. The Scottish First Episode Schizophrenia StudyVIII. Five year follow-up: clinical and psychosocial findings, *Br J Psychiatry* 1992;**161**:496-500.

306. Shepherd M, Watt D, Falloon I et al. The natural history of schizophrenia: a five-year follow-up study of outcome and prediction in a representative sample of schizophrenics, *Psychol Med* 1989;**Monograph Supplement 15**:1-46.

307. Leff J, Sartorius N, Jablensky A et al. The International Pilot Study of Schizophrenia: five-year follow-up findings, *Psychol Med* 1992;**22(1)**:131-45.

308. Goldstein JM, Kreisman D. Gender, family environment and schizophrenia, *Psychol Med* 1988;**18(4)**:861-72.

309. Seeman MV. Gender differences in schizophrenia, *Can J Psychiatry* 1982;**27(2)**:107-12.

310. Castle DJ, Abel K, Takei N et al. Gender differences in schizophrenia: hormonal effect of subtypes? *Schizophr Bull* 1995;**21(1)**:1-12.

311. Castle DJ, Murray RM. The neurodevelopmental basis of sex differences in Schizophrenia, *Psychol Med* 1991;**21**:565-575.

312. Russell AJ, Munro JC, Jones PB et al. Schizophrenia and the myth of intellectual decline, *Am J Psychiatry* 1997;**154(5)**:635-9.

313. Strauss JS, Carpenter WT Jr. The prediction of outcome in schizophrenia. II. Relationships between predictor and outcome variables: a report from the WHO international pilot study of

schizophrenia, *Arch Gen Psychiatry* 1974;**31(1)**:37–42.

314. Turner RJ, Gartrell JW. Social factors in psychiatric outcome: Toward the resolution of interpretive controversies, *Am Sociological Rev* 1978;**43(3)**:368–82.

315. Brown GW, Birley JLT, Wing JK. Influence of family life on the course of schizophrenic disorders: a replication, *Br J Psychiatry* 1972;**121**:241–58.

316. Erickson DH, Beiser M, Iacono WG et al. The role of social relationships in the course of first-episode schizophrenia and affective psychosis, *Am J Psychiatry* 1989;**146(11)**:1456–61.

317. Greenblatt M, Becerra RM, Serafetinides EA. Social networks and mental health: an overview, *Am J Psychiatry* 1982;**139**:977–84.

318. Abrahamson D. Institutionalisation and the long-term course of schizophrenia, *Br J Psychiatry* 1993;**162**:533–8.

319. McGlashan TH, Fenton WS. The positive-negative distinction in schizophrenia. Review of natural history validators, *Arch Gen Psychiatry* 1992;**49(1)**:63–72.

320. Engelhardt DM, Rosen B, Feldman J et al. Engelhardt JA. Cohen P. A 15-year followup of 646 schizophrenic outpatients, *Schizophr Bull* 1982;**8(3)**:493–503.

321. Zis AP, Goodwin FK. Major affective disorder as a recurrent illness: a critical review, *Arch Gen Psychiatry* 1979;**36(8 Spec No)**:835–9.

322. Tohen M. *Outcome in bipolar disorder. Doctoral dissertation*, Harvard University, Cambridge MA, 1988.

Index